I0897123

Embrace, Release, Heal

An Empowering Guide to Talking About, Thinking About, and Treating Cancer

Leigh Fortson

16pt

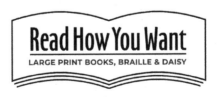

Read How You Want
LARGE PRINT BOOKS, BRAILLE & DAISY

Copyright Page from the Original Book

Published 2011

Book design by Dean Olson
Cover image © 2011 photolibrary.com

Printed in Canada

Library of Congress Cataloging-in-Publication Data

Fortson, Leigh.
    Embrace, release, heal : an empowering guide to talking about, thinking about, and treating cancer / Leigh Fortson.
        p. cm.
Includes bibliographical references.
    ISBN 978-1-60407-431-4
1. Cancer--Alternative treatment. 2. Cancer--Psychological aspects.
I. Title.
    RC271.A62F67 2011
    616.99'4--dc22
                                    2010037997

eBook ISBN 978-1-60407-456-7

10 9 8 7 6 5 4 3 2 1

TABLE OF CONTENTS

Praise for Embrace, Release, Heal

"Leigh Fortson has journeyed through territory where many will eventually go—the land of cancer. She has returned a very wise woman whose insights will empower anyone with this diagnosis. The stories and interviews in *Embrace, Release, Heal* are full of hope and meaning. I hope this inspiring book is widely read."

—Larry Dossey, MD, author of *The Science of Premonitions*

"America badly needs to expand its perspective on how to treat people with cancer. Limiting treatment to killing cancer cells without nurturing the person is like spraying roses without making sure that the soil they grow in contains the nutrients they require in order to thrive. *Embrace, Release, Heal* expands that perspective in a very personal, moving, and expert way. A must read if you or someone you love is dealing with cancer."

—Martin L. Rossman, MD, author of

Fighting Cancer from Within

"At last! In *Embrace, Release, Heal* we have testimony that proves that the healing of cancer involves the psychosomatic network of energy, mind, and spirit. Leigh Fortson is so courageous, not only for surviving her ordeal but also for standing up to the cancer docs who were shocked by the independent thinking and bold decisions that led to her recovery. This is a gripping, compassionate, and well-researched exposé that I hope will revolutionize cancer treatment in this country."

—Candace Pert, PhD, author of *Molecules of Emotion*

"Cancer patients face a bewildering array of emotions upon diagnosis, followed by a vast smorgasbord of treatment possibilities ranging from conventional medicine to alternative and complementary therapies. How does a patient cope with this onslaught, and how do they decide the course of their own therapy? With *Embrace, Release, Heal,* Leigh Fortson recounts her own

journey with cancer and gives us an extraordinary mix of personal anecdote, case studies, thoughtful analyses, and expert opinion in a positive and life-affirming fashion."
—William Bengston, PhD, author of
The Energy Cure

"*Embrace, Release, Heal* will radically expand your understanding of the cause of cancer and of how you can heal from this life-changing event. Leigh Fortson brings her unique perspective to the subject and emphasizes that cancer is not just a biological disease but something related to a bigger picture. She describes the impact of destructive thought patterns, emotional distress, and unhealthy habits—and shows how healing can happen when we replace destructive behaviors with a higher purpose."
—Ainslie MacLeod, author of
The Instruction and *The Transformation*

This book is dedicated to my husband,
Ed,
*whose enduring love and devotion
sustained me then and propels me now.*

***

*And to my children, **Tucker and Lyric,**
who inspire the depths of love,
the levity of delight,
and the wild humor necessary for this
crazy ride.*

FOREWORD

Infinite Possibilities

From the perspective of curative and preventive therapy, we have lost the war on cancer. Deaths from cancer are increasing. In 2008, there were 565,000 deaths in the United States alone. One in three people will get cancer in their lifetime. And few people know that solid tumors grow slowly for thirty years before they can be detected. We now have 17 million Americans walking around with cancer somewhere along the continuum from initiation of a cancer cell to detectable tumor.

In the "war" on cancer, we are fighting a losing battle for one simple reason: we are focusing on the wrong target. As a physician, I was trained to focus on the tumor: to burn, poison, or cut it out and then wait, watch, and pray for the cancer to stay at bay.

The problem with cancer is not the tumor, however, but the *garden* in which the tumor grows. In caring for a garden, if the weeds get too big, we pull them out—just as we do with cancer using conventional therapies. But then what? *Embrace, Release, Heal* is about the "then what." It's about the inexplicable, spontaneous remissions, cures of the incurable, about pioneering researchers, doctors, and patients exploring the edges of possibility and bumping up against a fertile science of how to tend our gardens.

The future of cancer care lies in the thinking and exploration found in this book. It provides a doorway of hope and possibility that rests in learning how to tend your own garden. The science supports this. But medical practice lags behind. Traditionally, we have focused on late-stage curative care, and in doing so, we have missed the thinking and the treatments focused on changing the underlying conditions that led to the cancer in the first place. Diet, lifestyle, thoughts, and environmental toxins all interact with our genes to change the landscape—or garden—of our health. We have been asking the wrong question about cancer. We have asked "what": What tumor do you have? What kind of chemotherapy, surgery, or radiation is needed for that tumor? What is your prognosis? Rather, we need to be asking "why" and "how": Why did this cancer grow? How can you change the conditions that feed and support cancer-cell growth? How did your garden become a host to such an invasive weed?

Surprisingly, scientific literature is abundant with evidence that diet, exercise, thoughts, feelings, and environmental toxins all influence the initiation, growth, and progression of cancer. If a nutrient-poor diet full of sugar, lack of exercise, chronic stress, persistent pollutants, and heavy metals can cause cancer, could it be that a nutrient-dense, plant-based diet; physical activity; changing thoughts and reactions to stress; and detoxification might treat the garden in which cancer grows? Treat the soil, not the plant. It is a foundational principle of sustainable agriculture, and of sustainable health.

In my oncology rotation in medical school, I asked my professor what percentage of cancer was related to diet. Expecting a gracious but insignificant nod to the role of diet as a cause of cancer, I was surprised when he said that 70 percent of all cancers were related to diet. The 2010 report from the President's Cancer Panel found that we have grossly underestimated the link between environmental toxins, plastics, and chemicals and cancer risk.[1] They have yet to acknowledge how thoughts, emotions, and overall stress impact that risk, but that acknowledgment is sure to come. The facts that gravitate around cancer support evidence that will motivate us all to take a deeper look.

Consider this fact: 16 percent of all cancers are new, primary cancers in patients who have had cancer, not recurrences. This means that people who have cancer are more likely to get a second and independent cancer. Could it be the garden? I recently saw a patient after her third cancer, wondering what she could do to prevent cancer rather than waiting around for another one.

Consider this fact: the lifetime risk of breast cancer for those with the "breast cancer gene," or BRCA1 or 2, is presently 82 percent and increasing every year. Before 1940, the risk of getting cancer for those with the cancer gene was 24 percent. What changed? Our diet, lifestyle, and environment—both physically and emotionally. Might these factors be a better place to look for answers to how to address our cancer epidemic?

Cancers arise from a disturbance in your physiological state. Addressing that disturbance is the foundation of future cancer care. This approach might be called milieu therapy. Rather than treating cancer per se, we treat the milieu in which cancer arises. And this is manageable: we can enhance immune function and surveillance through dietary and lifestyle changes, nutrient or phytonutrient therapies. We can facilitate our body's own detoxification system to promote the elimination of carcinogenic compounds. We can improve hormone metabolism and reduce the carcinogenic effects of too much insulin from our high-sugar and refined-carbohydrate diet, and help the detoxification of toxic estrogens through the modulation of diet and lifestyle and the elimination of hormone-disrupting xenobiotics or petrochemicals. We can alter how our genes are expressed by changing the inputs that control that expression—diet, nutrients, phytonutrients, toxins, stress, and other sources of inflammation. And we can focus on less divisive and more generative thoughts that, in turn, create more uplifting emotions—all good fertilizer for the soil in the garden of our body.

The future of cancer care must use medicine's understanding of the mechanisms of disease, as well as physiologic and metabolic balance, to design treatments that support and enhance normal physiology. The future of cancer care lies not in finding the best cocktail of chemotherapeutic agents, the right dose of radiation, or a new surgical technique, but in finding the right way to personalize treatment according to the individual imbalances in each person. This book contains the stories of the people—doctors and patients—who have paved the way. The pieces of the puzzle that hold the answers for cancer prevention and treatment are strewn about the landscape of medical science. They need only be assembled into a story that can guide clinical care. The time is ripe to accelerate this process. And this book begins the telling of the story of how to tend the gardens of our body, mind, and soul.

Mark Hyman, MD

Chairman, The Institute for Functional Medicine

August 1, 2010

ACKNOWLEDGMENTS

First, I offer my deep and heartfelt thanks to all who provided the stories and wisdom that have made this book a page-turner. Your contributions fill this thing with robust inspiration and will uplift anyone in need of hope. Without your willingness to share such intimate and remarkable stories, this book would not be in the hands of those who thirst for it. You are living proof that there are infinite possibilities for healing.

It takes a community to heal. I am blessed with a community of loving and generous friends all over the place. I throw buckets of gratitude into the faces of:

My Family

Eddie, for carrying me emotionally, spiritually, financially, and with irreverent humor.

Lyric and Tucker, for tolerating long retreats that enabled me to write without being asked to make dinner, go to the mall, or be picked up from tennis. Your light keeps my path bright.

Sandy Watson, my mom, for the unconditional love and willingness to do absolutely anything to help. Even from the nonphysical world, you give.

Angel LB, for your never-ending, totally loving support, and for several trips all the way from Germany to do laundry, make dinner, cheer up the kids, and help me frame the Journey so that I could cope. Oh—and for allowing me to write, rather than talk, during those rainy days on the Chesapeake Bay.

Lynn and John, for your presence in the kids' lives, your generosity, and your commitment to keeping life a creative venture.

Auntie Jaye, for welcoming me to Estes and the Denver condo, but mostly for the place you hold for me in your heart. It's ever more important now that Mom is gone.

The Georgia Fortsons, for constantly sending loving thoughts and prayers.

My Friends

Barbara Neighbors Deal, my agent, yes, but mostly a dear and trusted friend with whom I share great guffaws, spiritual perplexities, and a passion for fresh fruit and veggies.

Robin Gilman, for being the light during my darkest hours and for continuing to feed me spiritual gold. Here's to gourmet food, terribly expensive wine, and marveling at the wonder of our creations!

Andrea Leak, Rita Robinson, Carol Dix, Annalisa Sullivan, Dulce Bell-Bulley, Nova Sprick, Whitney Wogan, Leslie Schiller, Susan Walker, Jerry Sica, Colleen Scissors, David Gallagher, Joanna and Craig Little, Kohava Howard, Steph Carson, Susan Karbank, Ron Elliot, Barbara Mahoney, Kristin Lummis, Dana Hobika, Thomas Hunn, John Anglim, Kim Johnson, Doug Beube, Lynn Rae Lowe, and Zachariah Walker, for elevating the standard of what it means to be a true and great friend. Each of you supplied me with a unique piece of something I needed to break through to the other side.

Stella and Bill Pence, Brenda Krantz, Gib Johnson, Ed Rankin, Tony D'Agostino, Rose Shoshana, and Manfred Mueller, for demonstrating that long distances can't dissolve love, and for believing and investing in me even when you didn't necessarily know what I was doing.

Moira Magneson and Harry Brown, for your sharp editorial eyes that allowed me to send the manuscript to the publisher without being embarrassed, and for being really smart and really funny and making me feel that way, too.

Bing Lee, Dr. Louis DePalma, Kent Tompkins, Dr. Barre-Paul Lando, Dr. Bertrand and Roberta Babinet, Dr. Mark Hyman, Cindy Schmidt, Diana Shenkin, Christine Walcott, Anthony Bogart, Dr. Judith Boice, and Dr. Alex Gilmore, for being exceptional healers who treat the body, mind, and spirit. Thank you, thank you, thank you.

Robbie Levin, who gave me access to "the ranch" near Moab where some of my favorite parts of this book were written. Thanks also for being a supreme example of how to live a truly healthy lifestyle.

My devoted devil's advocate and angels team: Dr. Paul Preston, Dr. Barb

Zind, Dr. Lynda Hamner, Dr. Ken Scissors, Robbie, and Ed.

My Doctors and Nurses at the Regional Cancer Center and Wound Clinic

For all you did to help with my case, especially thanks to the nurses whose sincere care created a safety net that caught me in a series of freaked-out free falls. You are the fabric that keeps the good stuff in place.

My Colorado State University Office Mates

Nathan Moreng, Kellie Clark, and Rod Sharp, for covering for me when I was gone and keeping me in smiles when I'm there.

My Favorite Publishing House

Jennifer, Jaime, Haven, Shelly, Shanti, Tami, and all the great people at Sounds True, for showing what it means to act with integrity, generosity, and professionalism—all with the rare spirit of collaboration! One of the greatest days of my life was finding out that you wanted this book.

The Best Marketing Consultant

Tom Y. Sawyer of RSW Partners (rs wpartners.com), for your generous time and infinite wisdom.

Everyone Else

Finally, thanks to the many people not mentioned here who expressed love and provided sustenance during my Big Journey. You know who you are and how you gave so generously to me and my family. Thank you from the bottom of my heart.

INTRODUCTION

From the End to the Beginning

No pessimist ever discovered the secret of the stars, or sailed an uncharted land, or opened a new doorway for the human spirit.

HELEN KELLER

When my radiologist (we'll call him Dr. R.) told my husband, Ed, and me about my third cancer diagnosis, he was grim. Although Dr. R. is a very good man and a diligent and caring doctor, the seeds of hopelessness he planted within me that day were far more destructive than the centimeter-sized malignant tumor near my sciatic nerve that the biopsy had just confirmed.

"This doesn't bode well," he said, eyes staring at the chart on his lap. He explained that they couldn't use typical radiation because they had shot me with as much of it as my body could handle the first time I'd been down that road. Any more would do me in. Surgery wouldn't work either. I'd had surgery after my second diagnosis, and because the radiation from the year before had fried me so badly, it took nine long miserable months for my poor, compromised skin to heal. So no more radiation either. Apparently, for this new situation, chemo wasn't appropriate, which I was grateful to hear because, plain and simple, I don't like it, and I wasn't going to opt for it again.

"I'm pretty sure we can take care of the tumor that's there, but it's what's to come that ... it's what's to come..."

His words trailed off, but my imagination filled in the blanks. The pictures were paralyzing.

Ed and I left Dr. R.'s office gripping tightly to each other's hand. We were convinced that this diagnosis was the beginning of my end. We went to a park bench on that warm July day, and I wept between the bursts of terror that froze my body. Our children, Lyric and Tucker, eleven and thirteen years old, were the lights of our lives, and I couldn't bear leaving them motherless. They were my greatest concern and the source of a grief so deep I felt I would vomit if I had to contain it.

On that park bench, we talked in near grunts about how my husband would cope with being a single parent. His face was pale with shock, and he gripped my hand rigidly as though he were hanging on to a dissolving lifeline. We frantically turned the soil of our stiff minds and said aloud the names of family and friends who would inevitably step up to help raise our beautiful children. We knew they would do what they could to provide Lyric and Tucker with safe harbor after such a devastating loss.

Knowing that we would have to break the news to them about the recurrent cancer, we somehow managed the strength to stand, put one foot in front of the other, and make our way back to the car. As much as we wanted to protect them from the news until we ourselves could absorb the shock, there was no way either of us could hold back the intense emotions that shook us. My sister, Leslie, was visiting from

Germany, and my mother was scheduled to come for dinner that night. We would tell them all at once.

Lyric erupted into tears at the news. Sobbing, she kept saying, "I thought this was over! I thought we were done with this!" Tucker was stoic, shaking his head in disbelief. My mother cried silently as my sister held her hand and sent me love through the gaze of her tender, moist, brown eyes.

Finally, Lyric took a breath and asked, "Does God want you to die?"

After the previous two diagnoses, we had confidently told our kids that I would not die from the disease. This time, however, the only truthful answer was, "I don't know."

It was a long night of seemingly endless tears. Leslie wanted to do something helpful, so she set out to make a meal of comfort food: steak, mashed potatoes, vegetables, and dessert. As she prepared the steaks for the grill, she looked at me and said, "I know a woman who had brain cancer. Her brain was full of tumors. Everyone thought she was a goner. But she ate raw foods and did coffee enemas every day. She's fine now."

"How long ago did that happen?" I asked, thinking that the five-year survival rate I had been trained to believe in was an important marker.

"I don't know. Maybe twenty, twenty-five years ago."

Now a different seed was planted. I felt a physical sensation of something being uplifted and energized. "I could do that," I thought. "I *will* do that."

In that moment, I promised myself I would find a way clear. I would call that woman who had brain cancer twenty years ago and hear her story. I knew someone else who had healed herself from lung cancer. I'd call her too. I wiped away another round of tears and took a deep breath. Somehow, some way, I would find meaning and purpose and health. I would embrace my cancer and embrace the responsibility for my own wellness. I would release whatever was in my way of good health. By the grace of God, by my own tenacity, and by the infinite possibilities that are available to us *as long as we believe in them,* I would heal.

The Third Time's a Charm

Following the third diagnosis and during hours of contemplation, I knew something big had to change. The first diagnosis had put me through a brutal round of radiation and chemo. The second had resulted in three surgeries and a wound site that took nine long months to heal. This time I would do things differently, but I didn't know what or how. Should I start by eating raw foods?

The current cancer culture insists that diet doesn't matter and only chemo, radiation, and surgery can work. But they hadn't worked for me, and all I knew for sure was that going down that path again seemed insane. As Albert Einstein put it, the definition of insanity is "doing the same thing over and over again and expecting different results."

And so began the biggest adventure of my lifetime: to find new ways to treat my cancer. I was terrified at first.

I had no idea if any dietary changes, psychological inquiry, or alternative protocols would work. My doctors didn't believe in any of them, and some friends looked askance when they learned, for example, that I would become a raw foodist. I often teeter-tottered between sheer panic and doubt and blind faith. In my mind, however, I had no choice but to be open to everything—from hypnosis to cutting-edge treatments offered by an oncologist to herbs and enzymes suggested by a naturopath. I patently refused to buckle under the weight of the dismal prognosis delivered at the cancer center, and instead devoted myself to finding the center of my cancer so I could heal once and for all.

A few days after getting the bad news, Ed, Lyric, Tucker, and I spent a weekend in Breckenridge. It was one of those truly magical family trips where the kids didn't fight, the hotel was nice, the pool was big, and the food tasted good. Pinched in between all that were stolen moments between Ed and me, where we cried, held each other, and wondered how the hell we were going to make it through this.

When the weekend came to a close, I headed to Denver to see an oncology specialist. I left with an urgent need to keep my family together; to be there for my two exquisite, smart, and beautiful children; and to live beyond my fifty years. My gut twisted with anxiety about what treatments the specialist might suggest. Then it flip-flopped with excitement about trying new things, daring things that would define my adventure—stuff that the specialist in Denver surely wouldn't approve of.

As I turned onto I-70, it came to me: I would write a book! Surely other people wanted to find a new way of dealing with cancer, people like me who had tried all the conventional treatments without success. Or maybe there were people who wanted to bypass chemo, radiation, and surgery altogether. I simply couldn't accept that nothing else could work. I would write about what I found and share it with other seekers. Maybe, like me, there were people who hungered to know more about the possibility of spontaneous remission. I'd find people who had experienced it and write about them, too.

This idea invigorated me. I felt support from forces beyond this world. It was my way through.

Who knows the real truth behind the laws of God's universe? We can only hope that when the time is right, when conditions are such that change is the only option, a wave of invisible support will emerge from the heavens, and that which seemed so unlikely will come bounding through like a landslide of uncompromising opportunity.

By the time I sat down to write, I thought the book would be about some credible alternative cancer treatments, with a few good miracles thrown in. I thought I'd have to put an ad in the *New York Times* to find people who had healed cancer through alternative or spiritual means, but shortly into my journey, I quickly learned that these folks were *all over the place!* They could even be called fairly common! These were people written off by medical doctors after chemo, radiation, and surgery hadn't worked, simply because they knew no further options.

Nearly everyone I interviewed had been expected to die. As I heard their stories, my mind was slowly cleansed of doubt. I began to *believe* that it was possible to really and truly heal. These people had been in far worse shape than me, and now they were all thriving. Only a few still had signs of cancer, yet they were living completely functional lives, largely because of their new sense of purpose and because the treatments they chose were compatible with living a full and productive life.

Some of the people I spoke with regained health through alternative protocols; others simply *made the decision* to get well. Some gave credit to religion, faith, or spiritual dedication, while others spoke of what can only be known as grace. Most of them believe a bank of negative emotional turmoil contributed to the cause of their cancer. Likewise, they attribute much of their healing to creating an inner environment of love and forgiveness. All of them believe that we can heal ourselves or find effective treatments outside of the conventional medical paradigm.

These people enabled me to surrender my fears and replace them with hope. They were my guides, my angels. They made it possible for me to believe in my journey and ultimately my wellness. They are my heroes.

Their stories aren't the only things that inspired and educated me. So did interviews with naturopathic and alternative doctors and other health care practitioners who explained their innovative treatments—most of which medical doctors would readily dismiss. Since the Food and Drug Administration (FDA) doesn't condone most alternative cancer treatments, many of these doctors practice outside the United States. Despite what the FDA posits, the work of these practitioners is exciting, and they're enjoying a wide audience and good success.

Originally, I had not intended to include mainstream medical doctors and oncologists in this book, yet it became clear that to exclude them made no sense. Their stories are power-punched and just as promising as the others.

Plus, the healing journey is unique for everyone, and for those who choose to include conventional treatment in their menu of options (and many will), it's important to know which facilities offer the most holistic and progressive approaches. I've featured only a handful in this book, but thankfully, more and more are sprouting up across the country. (I've included additional references and information in the appendix. Also, check out my website for more: embracehealingcancer.com.)

I learned a great deal from these allopathic doctors, because they are some of America's greatest leaders and researchers in the cancer field. They understand the need to overhaul the cancer industry. They're working fiercely to reconstruct medical-school curriculums to include important dietary changes and emotional or spiritual support. Policies and politics are being scrutinized as well. Some of the docs are on a mission to clean up unethical conflicts of interest between medical researchers and the pharmaceutical industry, both of which essentially govern all allopathic medicine.

The politics of medicine and the profits that drive those politics are mind-boggling. We desperately need insiders like the doctors featured in this book in order to help change the parts of medicine that point to a faltering and corrupt business. Surprisingly, the only oncologist I interviewed perceives cancer as a multidimensional and even spiritual disease. Hearing his insights was like finding a pot of gold.

The book also includes stories of authors and experts who can explain just how extensive the relationship between our minds and bodies is. This isn't just a "connection," as it's commonly called. The two are actually *one organism.* For the purposes of healing, the implications of this union are huge. In a nutshell, if we dwell in (or repress) a world of conflict, stress, anger, and hatred, then the cells in our bodies and immune system respond accordingly and are weakened. At the same time, if the atmosphere we create contains positive qualities such as joy, playfulness, and peace—any of the attributes of love—then our cells and immune system are strong. Perhaps the best news is that we have the *choice* of which world we occupy. That choice—free will—is the very source of our personal power and authority.

We now have ample reason to follow the wisdom that spiritual masters and religious leaders from nearly every faith have been ministering to us since time began: Love your neighbor and yourself. Forgive. Find compassion. Be still. Give thanks. Create peace. The science behind these tenets promises good health in return.

The Emotional Map to Physical Well-Being

Given that science can now track the biological benefits of inner peace, isn't it time to give up the fight, the battle, *the war on cancer?* I know that goes against the grain of our shock-and-awe culture, but as the fatalities continue to mount, we have to admit the current medical battle strategy isn't working.

In writing this book, I've come to understand that what's really destroying us is our addiction to fighting—that the fight itself may indeed be part of why we get cancer. I also believe that when we surrender what often motivates a fight—anger, resistance, blame, judgment, resentment, or anything that eats away at us—then healing truly begins. In this context, surrender is actually the first and most powerful step toward wellness.

Giving up the fight doesn't mean relinquishing a healing protocol and being passive about what happens. In fact, healing requires a great deal of fortitude and due diligence. It means taking full responsibility for the quality of our lives and the choices we make.

On an emotional level, healing means releasing what tethers us to our sense of separateness, of being wronged, superior, inferior, lacking, and so on. It means giving up our habits of resistance and "against-ness," whether they are being directed toward our spouses, our bosses, our children, our parents, our friends, the government, corporations, or most especially, toward life, ourselves, or God.

Healing isn't a fight. Rather, healing is proactive and busy, contemplative and still. It is a process of educating ourselves about the options available and choosing the best fit. Healing also invites us to continually release every belief or habit that blocks us from living in peace. Healing is a holistic experience that inventories our physical and psychological lives, and then adjusts them if they are at odds with our purest intention to be well.

For many of us, calling upon invisible forces for help can serve to comfort, reassure, and surprise us with what some call miracles. Yet even atheists can experience these transformations, as long as they are willing to give up "against-ness" and dedicate themselves to peace and total wellness.

Healing from disease is about discovering the depth and breadth of who we really are, and then discovering what it means to live from our divine nature. When that happens, the entire world of possibilities presents itself anew.

The purpose of this book is to help empower those with cancer—or any type of degenerative illness—during a time when empowerment is in short supply. The book is a map that begins at a place of hope rather than fear. It invites you on a journey of peaceful exploration rather than asking you to muster the strength to wage war. Even if you choose to undergo conventional treatment—which I did—the book introduces strategies that bypass the "battle with cancer." Instead, it activates a relationship between your everyday self and your Greatest Self, a relationship in which true and lasting healing is possible. Without personal or emotional wholeness, our physical wellness is incomplete, and all the chemo and radiation in the world may not do a thing.

There is no guarantee that the map I've sketched out will lead you to being cancer free. But if you are true to yourself, if you can free yourself from what eats at you, I promise that you will find relief, peace, and love, and that the probability of being completely healed will be amplified.

I tell you the route I took and what I learned along the way. The stories in this book will provide inspiration and tools. But only you can bring your soul to this journey. Only you can determine how deeply you will go.

How to Use This Book

Read this book however you want. Reading straight through is good. Jumping around is fine. Each chapter title is noted by a single word that gives the essence or theme of the chapter. Pick and choose. No matter where you start, you'll be uplifted.

Stories help us make sense of madness. I include here both my own and the stories of other people who've had cancer. Most were told they would die. They didn't. After exhausting what conventional medicine had to offer, they walked away from the grisly prognosis and found another way. Some call it a miracle. I've come to believe it's just the way things work when we get out of our own way.

These stories will help inspire you to see the infinite possibilities that may be available to you, but that your doctor will likely dismiss. They reflect the truth that cancer can be effectively treated physically, emotionally, and spiritually through a different, more life-affirming paradigm than conventional medicine traditionally offers. These stories demonstrate why the conversation around cancer must be changed. If nothing else, I urge you to read all of them. Simply put, they are good medicine.

There are other stories here, too. The doctors and researchers unknowingly gave me hope for the medical system at large. It's heartening to know that there are exquisitely talented people working within the system and diligently trying to improve it. And they will. I trust you will find their information useful and enriching.

Finally, the authors, experts, and spiritual perspectives of the people I spoke with can enlighten you to the power within. While the crosshairs of collapse are centered on our current health care system, it's imperative to finally acknowledge that *the mind plays perhaps the most significant role* in our journey toward wellness. In the existing cancer culture, our state of mind is given little, if any, responsibility for the reasons we may get cancer in the first place or for potentially catapulting us into complete and final healing. We're at the point where it's practically impossible to separate the scientific from the spiritual, as both are playing out the same stories—through us. At last, cutting-edge scientists are able to show us how.

Each interview can be read as a new way of talking about, thinking about, and treating cancer. I include differing points of view, trusting that one or more of them will speak directly to you and light the way for your own unique path to wholeness and healing.

Although I emphasize diet, the power of the mind, spiritual prowess, and some alternative treatments, I won't tell you to cancel your next appointment with the oncologist. Instead, once you know there are other options, I simply ask that you look within and determine for yourself what is the best possible treatment for your condition. By looking within, by accessing your own unique and personal expression of wisdom, and by trusting your own authority, you will come to know yourself and what is best for you.

A good creed to keep in mind: "Cancer is a word, not a sentence." I believe this, and I hope to take it at least one step further by suggesting that cancer is an opportunity not only to live life fully, but also to empower ourselves to heal on every level.

Typically, people who are diagnosed with cancer are taught to believe in limitations rather than in possibilities. Yet by opening our minds, by exploring and loving the deepest parts of ourselves, and by negotiating our own path with the light of the inherent power within, we can quickly realize, with great shouts of joy, that we are boundless. Indeed, we *are* the possibilities.

***

Note: There is no single point of view presented in this book. I do not necessarily agree with the treatments or opinions of all the people I interviewed. Likewise, the doctors, patients, and authors cited in the book do not necessarily agree with one another, nor with everything I offer to my readers.

All growth is a leap in the dark, a spontaneous unpremeditated act without the benefit of experience.

HENRY MILLER

CHAPTER 1

My Story

Life is not the way it's supposed to be.
It's the way it is. The way you cope
with it is what makes the difference.
VIRGINIA SATIR

My story is about change.

I was living, by any standard, a good life. I had survived the tough times in my marriage and was happy with my husband. I had two smart, funny, healthy, and engaging kids. I loved my job, lived in a pretty house, enjoyed an uplifting spiritual life, and had a great group of friends. But all of that changed.

I went from living a good life to living a great life. I went from being unaware of the extent of the stress I carried, the degree of fear I harbored, and how many dreams I had abandoned to the awareness I have now.

Now I respond quickly to relieve stress. Now I have a new understanding of the source and role of fear and how it can awaken our greatest opportunity to heal. Now I am deeply grateful for all that I have, and for the most part, I dwell in feelings of joy and awe. Now my dreams are inspired and driven by the ongoing discovery of ways and reasons to trust in this magnificent, painful, rich, mysterious, challenging, brilliant, and benevolent ride we call life.

All because of cancer.

Episode One: Physical

My first diagnosis came in 2006, after I struggled for years with a painful hemorrhoid. My doctor, Jane, checked it out during routine visits, but when I requested that it be surgically removed, she agreed.

Anal cancer didn't get much press before the beautiful television star Farrah Fawcett was diagnosed just weeks after I was. It was embarrassing to have cancer of the ass, and although I tried to laugh at the jokes my friends bandied about for the sake of levity, I was mortified. The prognosis, at least, was good.

"Don't max out your credit cards," the lovely Indian surgeon told me. "Ninety percent of anal cancers are cured through chemo and radiation."

That happy statistic didn't matter. I couldn't wrap my mind around the idea of doing those treatments. It was both terrifying and outrageous. I was healthy, for God's sake! I exercised, wrote books about alternative medicine and nutrition, and only occasionally indulged in fast food. Having cancer was not "me." I felt confused, frightened, and hopeless.

My husband, Eddie, held me. Then he looked deeply into my eyes. At first he said nothing, just allowed a small smile to lighten his face. His eyes penetrated mine so deeply that I thought I caught a glimpse of eternity.

"We'll make it through this," he promised and pulled me back into the warmth of his embrace. He then reminded me that I could look into alternatives.

Strangely, that hadn't yet occurred to me. After being given the diagnosis, I was told what to do. I was given the name of an oncologist and radiologist whom I would visit, and they would design the protocol. There was no discussion about options; no mention of diet, exercise, or the mind-body connection; and nothing about alternative cancer treatments that might be available. In my state of shock, I absorbed it all without question. Like all good patients, I listened, nodded, and agreed to the plan. Like most patients, I felt scared witless, because just the word "cancer" delivers the very real blow that your time on this planet could be cut short.

After Ed's prompting, I spoke to a German doctor whose protocol sounded noninvasive and promising. It would deplete all of our savings, and I would need to make frequent visits to Cologne, where he practiced. My sister, Leslie, lived in Germany, and it didn't sound terribly unreasonable for me to travel there for treatment. After further discussions, the straight-talking doctor said, "Listen, they have good luck with radiation and anal cancer. Stay there. Be close to your family. Save your money." It was the rational choice, but every ounce of my body resisted it.

Dr. O., the oncologist, was a gentle, bright, young, upbeat man and a good listener with a great sense of humor. He explained that the type of chemo I would do was a low-dose, low-toxicity variety. I wouldn't lose my hair. They would surgically implant a port into my chest so I could be hooked up to the chemo five days a week. I would carry the chemo in a fanny pack, and a tube would travel under my shirt to the port that would continuously feed me the drug.

Dr. R., the radiologist, was a quiet, serious man, but someone I trusted from the start. Radiation treatments were scheduled for five consecutive days, and as with the chemo, I'd have weekends off. It was a six-week protocol.

***

Eddie held my hair back as I vomited. It was the first day of chemo. He grabbed the prescription Dr. O. had given him in case of this kind of violent reaction and brought me the $400-per-pill meds designed to help. They did. I had good health insurance from my job at Colorado State University, and I was extraordinarily blessed for that.

My mind, however, would not stop spinning. I had adopted a belief system that says we create our own reality, yet at the time, I couldn't see my way to that. I never would have given myself cancer. I was confused and overwhelmed. This diagnosis and treatment completely stripped me of my understanding of who I was, and I no longer had any clue what to believe spiritually.

I began working with an intuitive but scientifically schooled man from Boulder named Bertrand Babinet. He urged me to take homeopathic tinctures and specific vitamins during the treatment. He worked closely with a progressive oncologist in Florida, and she e-mailed him a list of things that would help with side effects.

Drs. O. and R. and the cancer center's pharmacist were opposed to me taking the tinctures and vitamins "in case any of them might block the effectiveness of the treatments." Bertrand promised there would be no contraindications, but against my instincts, I gave in to my physician's advice.

The third week of treatment slammed me down. I could no longer leave the house because of fast and wicked bouts of diarrhea. I was increasingly fatigued and nauseated. By the end of that week, the mucous membranes in my crotch—and believe me, there are many—were purple, swollen, and burning. By week four, I could no longer use toilet paper. My husband bought a baby-bottle warmer so I could warm the spray bottle that I used for cleaning myself. The pain took my breath away. Unable to sit and barely able to walk, I spent most my time prone in bed.

Life as I knew it was over, but life went on just the same. Friends brought dinner almost nightly. My mother did laundry, washed dishes, and helped the kids with homework. One friend gave me regular foot massages, while a generous neighbor walked my dogs. Leslie flew in from Germany, did household chores, gave backrubs, reassured the kids, and drove me to my daily radiation sessions. Perhaps her most valuable contributions were holding my hand as I cried and offering her best ideas on how to find the strength to endure.

I spoke to Bertrand almost weekly. He held me by the spiritual hand and sensed with alarming accuracy what was going on inside me. He helped me identify all the parts within me that were going through this: the child, the protector, the rebel. He helped me make sense of my confusion, and on days when there was nothing but bleak darkness, his comfort and wisdom carried me to the light.

My mother called me well into my treatments and said, "I'm going to buy a tree. I'm going to plant it and put a plaque under it with your name on it."

The news jarred me. "Mom, you do that *after* someone dies, not before, and I'm not going to die."

She said, "There are people who have parties before they die. Everyone gets together to celebrate the person so they can know just how much people loved them."

I paused. "Are you suggesting we have a party?"

"No, I'm just telling you that's what some people do."

Like most everyone, my mother was caught in the web of fear that the cancer culture drags through the material of our minds. When you get diagnosed, you can tell which people assume you will die and which are rooting for you. You learn to avoid the ones who are already writing sympathy cards to your family, and you keep company only with those who are willing to watch silly movies with you and talk about taking a trip together next year. But I couldn't push my own mother out of my life. She had a heart of gold, and I needed and loved her.

After I got over being angry with her for wanting to memorialize me in my fourth week of treatment, I awakened to the fact that she was a woman whose daughter had cancer. She was terrified of losing her child. She was watching her baby wither away, and she didn't know how to deal with it. Unfortunately, I was no comfort to her. I could barely comfort myself because I didn't know how to deal with it either.

Not long after our conversation, she planted a tree in her back yard. Then she had a mild stroke, and there was nothing I could do to help.

One day, I lay in bed and just prayed that I could cope—just cope, that's all. In moments when the pain was unbearable, I would shuffle to the bathroom and submerge myself under the shower until the warm water became cold. It was the only place I found relief. I couldn't allow the water to splash directly on the burns, but the drops that flowed down my back and stomach found the crevices where I was swollen, and the moisture of the water soothed me for a second or two, maybe three. Tears streamed down my face, mixing with the tepid water.

"What happened?" I kept asking myself. "What happened to my life?"

I no longer knew who I was. I was no longer strong, no longer active, no longer light. I no longer knew what to think, because I had thought that I was healthy. I no longer knew that tomorrow would come. I no longer felt the presence of God. The "me" I had been was simply no longer.

Eddie kept the house together, worked extra hours to cover the bills, and shopped for groceries. He brought me smoothies and stroked my hair. He looked into my eyes, offering a glimpse of eternity once again.

"All those things," he once said in a near whisper, "those little things that used to bother me about you, they're gone." He smiled.

"Yeah," I replied, "they're gone from me, too."

"They're nothing. They're meaningless. How did we make them so big?"

I shook my head. It was true. I felt completely free of criticism or judgment toward him. I felt only a constant flow of adoration, appreciation, gratitude, and ever-deepening love.

"You are the strongest person I've ever known," he told me with conviction.

I didn't feel strong. But I did feel loved—deeply, purely, and fiercely loved—by him; by my mother and sisters; by the people who sent me cards, flowers, and food; by my phenomenal community of friends who kicked in to keep the lives of my kids normal; and by my dog, Tika.

Tika, a border collie mix, was—and still is—my devoted companion. Ed began to sleep in a different room because my sleeping patterns were so erratic, but Tika stayed by my side day and night. Her loyal and intense brown eyes stared compassionately at me as I screamed at the God I no longer trusted, as I cursed my life for falling to shreds, or in quiet moments when I stroked her soft ears more for my sake than for hers. I asked her questions that neither man nor beast could answer. Her tail would wag, and somehow, it would fan a smile from me.

At the peak of my suffering, a dear friend sent me an audio book by Jean Shinoda Bolen called *Close to the Bone: Life-Threatening Illness and the Search for Meaning*. The title scared me. I couldn't fathom that I had a life-threatening disease.[1]

One morning, as I fought with the sheets to try and free myself of pain,

I decided to listen. I hazed in and out of the book until the author told a story about how when people are very sick and facing their mortality, they often experience something similar to the mythological character of Persephone.

Persephone was kidnapped and taken from her mother by Hades, the god of the Underworld, where he kept her. No one knew where she went. She didn't know if she would ever surface and smell the flowers on the topsoil again. Her mother cried and cried. The myth went on, but at that moment something finally clicked.

I too had been kidnapped. I too was in the Underworld. I didn't know if or how I would ever resurface again, but at least now I knew where I was. It comforted me somehow, in some way, because that story gave me a context for where I was—in the Underworld with Persephone—and knowing that enabled me to sleep through the night.

On the Friday of my fifth week of treatment, I told Dr. O. that I could no longer continue with treatment. The burns were too much. I asked for his blessing.

He smiled compassionately and said that he would have a look at the burns. When he did, he ended with, "You're just where we want you. If you were my mother, my sister, or my wife, I'd say the same thing. One more week, and it'll all be over."

The following Monday, my dear friend Andrea, a nurse, drove me to the cancer center. I was exhausted from the pain. It was much worse than it had been the previous Friday. We parked. I stared straight ahead and shook my head at the thought of doing more. I opened the door and slowly inched my legs to the side so I could put my feet on the pavement. The moment my feet landed on the cement, I was certain.

"I'm not doing anymore," I told her over my shoulder. "I'm done."

"OK," she agreed. "You're done."

I sat in Dr. O.'s office, waiting for his nurse to prepare the port so I could get hooked up to the chemo tube, although this time I wouldn't be doing that. She walked in with Dr. O. following behind. I told them the news.

Dr. O. looked puzzled. He had just checked me days earlier.

"It's so much worse," I said. "I can't do it anymore."

He told me to lie back, and he'd have another look. When he saw my burns, his eyes widened, and he recoiled just enough before he caught himself. I knew he would agree to stop.

"OK," he said. "You're done."

Radiation works that way. It doesn't burn a little more with each treatment. It burns more by the hour. The burns had increased exponentially from the previous Friday at 5:00p.m. to that Monday at 8:00a.m.

After he left, his nurse leaned into me and said, "It's barbaric, this treatment. Barbaric." She was one of many nurses at the cancer center for whom I held deep affection. Their good and loving hearts counteracted the toxicity of the chemo that bullied my veins. They made it possible for me to show up every day without losing my mind.

Next, it was time to tell Dr. R. that I was finished. Since radiation was his thing, I figured he would be more resistant. When his nurse checked me in, I began to cry. I was afraid Dr. R. would insist. She took my hand and said, "It's your body. You can do whatever you want."

It's easy to forget that in a cancer center.

It was Halloween, and Dr. R., a typically quiet and private man, entered the office wearing camouflage army fatigues. "Don't shoot me," I half chuckled, "but I don't want to do any more radiation. Dr. O. agrees that I'm finished."

He cocked his head with curiosity, checked out the damage, and said, "I've seen worse."

I was aghast. I couldn't imagine worse. He urged me to do five more treatments, even compromising by allowing me to do three treatments that week and two the next. He wanted me to complete the full six-week course, but radiation continues to burn even on days without treatment. I shook my head no. I was firm. Reluctantly, he understood.

Andrea bought me an aloe vera plant and told me to put the juice of the leaves directly on the burned tissue. It was the best gift I'd ever been given. It worked, and I healed within about two weeks—enough, at least, so that I could walk without bowing my legs and taking baby steps.

Soon I would surface. Soon I would leave the Underworld. Soon I would be back in the spring of life. I could leave all of it behind. I could forget about it forever.

As the months went by, my body was getting better by the day, but emotionally I was still out of shape. The more I took on a normal life, the more I decided this whole cancer business of mine was a fluke. I didn't like to talk about having cancer, and I never called myself a cancer survivor. I didn't like identifying with the cancer world in any way whatsoever. Somehow, God had made a mistake and drawn my number when someone else was supposed to get it. But once you've been diagnosed with cancer, you're branded, and even if you want to let it go, others won't.

Several months after I was through with treatments, I was at a party at my mother's house. A woman I had never met came up to me and said, "Are you Leigh?" I nodded. "Oh my God!" she wailed, putting her heavy arm on my shoulder. "Do you have any idea what you've put us through?"

I knew exactly what she was talking about, but I didn't want to give her any more fuel to fan her dramatic flames. "No," I said flatly.

"Well, it's been hell," she said.

I discreetly removed her arm and said, "It's over now." And I walked away.

I was diligent about getting my body back on track. I committed to a regimen of acupuncture, massage, healing touch therapy, and chiropractic care. My naturopathic doctor gave me a homeopathic tincture to help remove the radiation from my body. I was determined to get out of the cancer jungle and the feelings of utter hopelessness that had plagued me that year. I could soon act as though it had never even happened.

Episode 2: Emotional

One year after my first diagnosis, I was convinced that the rectal bleeding I was experiencing was from internal hemorrhoids. I refused to believe differently. But when the pain set in, I decided it was time for a check-up. I was terrified.

"There's something here," Dr. R. said as he examined me. His face had suddenly paled. "I think it's a recurrence."

Only a biopsy would confirm it, so the nurses hooked me up with the newest, youngest, most progressive gastrointestinal (GI) doc in town. A few days later, I was in his office.

"I would be very surprised if it's cancer," he told me reassuringly. "A few months ago, you had a normal CT scan, and there was nothing. Cancer doesn't just show up overnight. If this is cancer, I'll have to change my whole way of thinking."

During the biopsy, I regained consciousness on the table as the GI doc performed the last part of it. I was on my side, facing the television screen where I could see his instrument plucking away at an angry, irritated, concave mass.

"What's that?" I asked groggily.

"We'll talk later."

I'm sure he thought I wouldn't remember a conversation while under sedation, but I still see that image clearly in my mind. In that moment, I knew it was cancer.

It was a few days before Labor Day weekend when we heard the definitive news that the disease had moved up the anal canal and was now embedded in the wall of my rectum. I was a graduate of anal cancer, and now I was signed up for rectal cancer. This time, treatment would mean surgically removing my anus, my rectum, and part of my sigmoid colon. I would need a colostomy bag. It would be irreversible.

"But," said Dr. R., with visible empathy in his eyes, "it will save your life."

The friendly GI doc would now have to rethink everything he knew. And so would I.

After my first diagnosis, Ed and I had promised the kids that radiation and chemotherapy would cure the cancer. Now it was time to tell them it had not.

We did our best to deliver the news in an upbeat manner. This time, we're going to cut it out! This time, there won't be any chemo or radiation to make me sick! This time, I'll be better in a matter of weeks! In fact, Dr. O. told me with all confidence that I'd be back on my bike within a month after the operation! No big deal!

And then we told them what a colostomy was.

Around that same time, Farrah Fawcett also had a recurrence of cancer.

Dr. O. and Dr. R. both recommended a surgeon in Denver whom they believed was well suited for me, which probably meant he'd sit patiently through all my questions and indulge my often off-color humor.

Before leaving for Denver, I visited the ostomy nurse in Grand Junction, where I live. She would determine exactly where the stoma would be located according to the types of clothes I wore and the contours of my body.

Eddie went with me to see her. Robin was a cheerful, attentive, and positive woman. I immediately felt safe with her. As she examined my abdomen, surveying my skin and posture, she made a black mark on my abdomen and said, "I think this is just the right spot."

I started to cry. I couldn't accept the fact that my intestines were going to be sticking out of my stomach. I couldn't bear the idea of defecating into a bag. I was overwhelmed with fear.

She took my hand, "You go ahead and cry. You *should* cry. This is scary, I know, but you're going to make it through this. I'll be here for you no matter what you need. I'll teach you whatever you need to know. You can call me anytime. I know it seems awful, but you'll get used to it. And you'll live a good and happy life."

Her deep, compassionate brown eyes held mine, touching me very deeply. I believed her. She smiled. Her hand held mine tightly, while Eddie's hand cupped my knee. I was surrounded by angels.

Tucker and Lyric had to go through so much at such young ages, but there was nothing I could do to change that. My mother had fully recovered from her stroke, and leaving the kids in her loving care was the best I had to offer. It had been almost exactly a year since I had begun radiation and chemo. Now my beloved husband was driving me to Denver so I could have my bowels rearranged.

I kept the tears at bay until we exited the subdivision. It was a quiet ride over the Continental Divide, Eddie holding my hand almost the entire way.

The hospital was brand spanking new—and enormous—with shiny glass windows that shimmered and towered over the broken-down neighborhoods that skirted it. We dropped our stuff at a nearby hotel and had a quick meeting with the surgeon, Dr. D. He was nice, nerdy, and very present. He answered my questions thoroughly, but didn't know what to do when I started to cry. It seemed like he needed an explanation. I recalled Robin's promises for a good and happy life when she marked my tummy for the stoma placement. I recalled how she had acknowledged my fears.

"This is scary," I grunted.

Dr. D. nodded, saying nothing for a moment. Then, as though remembering that communication helps, he said, "You'll be sore for a few days, maybe a week. But it will all be fine within a month."

Trying to keep the conversation moving forward, I asked him about doing a skin flap. One of the doctors I had interviewed a few weeks earlier had urged me to have the procedure done. It had something to do with helping the wound heal faster. Dr. D. shook his head.

"That's an additional operation that requires a different kind of doctor. I don't feel the need for it. I'm not sure why anyone would suggest it."

I accepted his response. No one else had mentioned it either.

Lovemaking that night was slow, intimate, and awash in deep, salty sorrow.

We arrived at the hospital at 5:00a.m. and checked in along with the rest of the herd. There must have been twenty other people there for one kind of operation or another.

"Well, you're about to become a freak," I heard something inside me say. I shivered. Eddie held me until a nurse with a clipboard called my name.

I was taken back to a "stall" where only flimsy curtains separated me from the next patient. The nurses and techs asked routine questions and began prepping me for the operation. They covered my back with adhesive tape so that they could give me an epidural. The more they worked on me, the more frightened I became.

It was my turn to be wheeled away. Eddie leaned in to me and gave me those eyes that promise forever, no matter what. He whispered in my ear and said he'd be there the second I awoke.

I wrapped my arms around him. I couldn't release the familiar warmth, comfort, and breadth of his body. It had provided me with so much strength in the past year, so much hope. His love was all I could count on. He was all I could fasten myself to. My world was slipping away, but he was steady. I gripped on to him tightly until at last he peeled himself away. "You have to go now, my darling. It'll be OK. It'll be OK."

Three nurses wheeled me down a long yellow-white hallway. I was going to lose a body part, one you use every day. I was going to be a freak. I leaned up on my elbows and looked at one of the nurses. "What happened to my life?" I cried. "What happened to my life?" My eyes darted at the trio of surprised nurses. I sobbed, spitting out my question over and over. In a moment I didn't notice, a mask was placed over my face, and everything I could discern disappeared.

My eyes opened to Eddie's sweet, concerned smile. He stroked my forehead. "Hello my darling, you made it through," he said. "Look who's here."

Beautiful, charismatic Manfred had flown in from Los Angeles the previous night to be with Eddie. They peered down at me. Manfred grinned warmly and told me in his thick German accent that I looked pretty. I held his hand, feeling deep gratitude that he had come. My beloved had been my rock, but he needed support, too.

I perceived that the room I occupied was small and somehow different. There were no windows, no medical instruments, no tables, no chairs. "Is this the recovery room?" I asked with parched lips and a tongue stiff with dryness.

The big fancy hospital had overbooked its reservations. The recovery room, it turned out, was full to capacity. I was in a storage closet. But I was lucky, because there were others outside the door, lining the halls. I figured that I had gotten special treatment because they were afraid I would start wailing again. The squeaky wheel and all. Lucky me, indeed.

"See what good things you attract?" Eddie asked. "You get the closet!"

I tried to laugh, but my mouth felt like cracked dirt. I begged for ice chips, and someone finally brought me some. I fell asleep with the welcome feeling of moisture in my mouth.

A day later, I was given a private room. A day after that, my back began to itch—really badly. With a good dose of self-disdain, I realized I had neglected to tell the nurses who had prepped me for the operation that I was highly allergic to adhesive tape. My back was covered in tape, and I was breaking out in festering hives.

Dr. D. escorted an entourage of medical students on his rounds. When I complained of the unbearable itching, he gingerly turned me over on my side. He removed the tape. The students were mesmerized. Maybe they had never seen anything like it. As my stay at the hospital progressed, the hot-tempered rash on my back became as much of an intrigue as the wound site in my butt, which wasn't behaving quite as it should.

Emotionally, something had shifted. I wasn't as frightened. The operation was over, and I was alive. I would be able to function, even with that thing sticking out of my belly. It was actually kind of pretty. Some people call it a rosebud. I saw why.

Still, I was a long way from being at peace. I was weak, unable to walk, suffering unbelievable itching on my back, and unable to move myself from the hips down. And I was deeply, gut-wrenchingly sad.

Each morning, a spiritual counselor visited me. He was young and receptive. Each morning, he asked how I was, and I would quietly cry.

"Why do you think this kind of stuff happens?" I asked, hoping that one of these mornings he would provide an answer that would kick-start my faltering spiritual life. "I don't know," he answered honestly. "I really don't know."

Each morning as I cried, he passed me tissues. There were few words. He would sit with me for a good half hour. After his last visit, I found that I did feel closer to the God I had believed in so devotedly before my first diagnosis. This young man was simply present with me, and his presence reminded me that presence is sometimes all that we need and all that we really have.

Presence and love.

I had never met Bertrand, the man who had been a spiritual advisor over the phone, but he and his wife, Roberta, came to visit. I was in a drug fog, but I was aware enough to see their faces. Bertrand sat next to me and did nothing more than hold my hand. I felt the warmth coming through my hand and up my arm. Bertrand's presence gave me a new feeling of calm.

My cousin's wife, Kim, whom I had spent very little time with, came to the hospital one day and massaged my feet. She had practiced healing therapies, and I was so deeply relaxed and soothed by the massage that I couldn't find the words to thank her for her presence in that moment.

My Auntie Jaye came to visit several times, bringing me good food and a cheerful smile. My sisters both visited. Herbert, an old and dear friend, whose wife had died a year prior, brought me sweatpants that I could wear on the drive home, since my jeans were too tight for my extremely sore arse.

Love showed up in so many faces.

After eight days in the hospital, it was time to go home. There was no way I could sit down for the four-hour drive, so we borrowed a van from Whitney, a dear old friend who lived in Boulder. She delivered it complete with a sleeping bag, pillows, and a pile of feather blankets on the floor in back so

I could be prone for the duration. I felt Whitney's presence in the warmth of the blankets.

The doctors gave me an extra dose of painkillers and something to soothe my nerves. It was a strange drive. My body swayed back and forth with the curving mountain roads. I watched the clouds overhead and the pine trees on the mountainsides as we passed. I was in a dreamlike state, unable to sleep or sit up and talk with Eddie.

About an hour from the hospital, I had to go to the bathroom. We were in a small tourist town, and we stopped at the visitor's center. Eddie helped me out of the side door of the van. I was thin, fragile, and weak. A tour bus had arrived just before us, and a crowd of mostly white-haired people milled about. When they saw me, they stopped talking, looked at me with soft eyes, smiled gently, and made way for me to pass.

Eddie led me to the line at the restroom. The person at the end of the line said, "Go ahead of me," and so did the person before her, and so did the person ahead of her. Everyone in line stepped back and urged me to the front. Each person in this line of elderly people—some with hearing aids, some with thick glasses and pupils white with age, some with canes, some with limps and arthritic hobbles—waved their hand, signaling me to go ahead of them. I will never forget both the generosity of their hearts and the feeling that I was older and sicker than they were. I was so much more in need than these people who could have been twice my age.

When I got home, the love of my children, my mother, my sisters, and our dogs swarmed me. It was good to be away from the war zone of the hospital, the tubes and beeps and horrible alarms of the IV pole, the smells and manufactured food. I was home at last.

The anger I had maintained after my first diagnosis had dissolved. Instead, I was vulnerable. I grew ever more humble. I was unable to function normally because the surgery site left an open wound the size of an orange that was not healing. I was at risk for infection, and if I got one, it could make me very ill or even kill me. I was told not to submerge myself in water. I couldn't sit. I couldn't bend over. I had lost considerable weight. I was slow in body, but soft in spirit.

Eddie, my mother, and both my sisters attended to me. When I was in the shower and my sister Lynn got on her hands and knees to shave my legs, for the first time I saw something uniquely beautiful: I was forced to be on the receiving end. I had never liked to ask for help, but now I didn't have to; it was a given that I needed it. My circumstances had mixed up the dynamic of my nature, which was to be the capable one, the one who helps, the one who organizes and produces. It quieted my proactive personality, and rather than being the one who took care of business, I had no choice but to be in the loving hands of those who took care of mine. Being on the receiving end was a whole new twist, and in certain ways, it was liberating. I had to let go. I had to learn to accept, rather than resist, my life as it was.

A week later, Mom had another stroke. Again, I could do nothing to return the love and attendance she had so generously bestowed upon me.

Dr. D. ordered a home-health nurse to visit me three days a week. Betsy was feisty, outspoken, and sun weathered; married to a womanizing cowboy; and constantly worrying about her two bull-riding sons. I liked her spirit, but she was loud and overly talkative. I was in a quiet place, and I wasn't sure if our union would work.

On about her third visit, I was depressed. The wound site wasn't improving. The stitches had fallen out, and the area was wet and weepy. I had the unpleasant chore of changing the dressing several times a day. On her visits, Betsy would clean out the inner part of the wound.

I lay on my side while she checked it out. "This ain't right," she said. "You gotta get it looked at."

I stood up and protested with tears. I couldn't travel back to Denver to see Dr. D. because I couldn't endure the trip. I was no longer using my doctor, Jane, or the Indian surgeon who had conducted the hemorrhoidectomy. Both had become too emotionally involved and insulting when I chose to use Dr. R.'s approach to follow-up exams rather than their approach. Who would I go to? What would I do?

Betsy was empathetic. "I can order up some antidepressants for you. They'll help."

"What?" I asked, appalled at her suggestion. "Those are for people who don't know why they're depressed. I have *reason* to be depressed! I've had two cancer diagnoses. My mom just had a second stroke. I have a gouge in my ass the size of a tennis ball, I have no doctor, I'm in constant pain, I can't sit down, and the wound is getting worse. Don't you think I have the *right* to be depressed? Don't you think I should just *go through this* because it's actually *normal* to be depressed under these circumstances?"

Still crying, I stuffed my dresser drawers with clean clothes and then slammed them shut.

Betsy was slack-jawed. Slowly, she nodded and placed her hands on her hips. "You're right, you know that?

People just swallow them pills for any damn thing. And here you are with good reason, and you won't. You're one strong woman. And you know what? You're going to make it through this because of that, and I'm going to stand by you all the way. Now let's get a fucking doctor on your case."

After what seemed like hundreds of phone calls, I was finally advised to see the local wound specialist. We'll call him Dr. W. By then, Robin, the ostomy nurse, had become a close friend. She told me to be clear and ask Dr. W. questions because his strength is surgery, not necessarily communication.

When Dr. W. arrived in the exam room, he shook my hand but looked at Eddie, not me. Then he and Alice, his nurse, spoke in a language that neither Eddie nor I could decipher. Alice would say something in half sentences, and Dr. W. would often answer with a single word.

I rolled over and pulled apart my cheeks so he could assess the damage. He peered and tilted his head this way and that, saying nothing, but breathing loudly.

"Can you fix me?" I asked.

There was no reply.

"Can you heal me?" I pleaded.

"Well," he said, rolling backward on his wheeled stool. "That's the objective."

I began to ask questions. Alice answered in short snippets of sentences that she would start and then restart. Dr. W. headed for the door.

"You're not leaving, are you?" I blurted, sitting up on my side.

He looked surprised. "I was planning to, yes."

I recalled Robin's sage advice and said, "Oh no, you don't. I have questions for you."

Alice laughed, and Dr. W. acquiesced, "Oh? OK, what?"

He stood at the door with one foot in the hall. I shot my questions at him. He answered them sometimes clearly, sometimes vaguely. Alice would interpret or embellish. When I was done, I thanked him.

"Can I go now?" he smiled with a sly eye.

"Yes, you may go."

"You're not going to shoot me?"

"Not anymore," I answered, grinning.

He vanished. Alice was glowing. "He'll get you healed," she promised. "He's a really good doctor. He just doesn't like to say he can do it, but he will."

Her sparkling eyes warmed my soul. I believed her.

I saw Dr. W. three times a week in addition to the three weekly visits from Betsy. He may not have been a great communicator, but Dr. W. had a wonderful, cunning sense of humor, and it wasn't long before we spiced up our visits with playful bantering and crass jokes that only a major wound in the derriere can inspire.

I was crammed with every imaginable type of gauze and healing ointment. I affectionately referred to these treatments as "stuffing the turkey." I changed the dressing three to four times a day in an attempt to keep the bandages clean and dry. The only way I could manage the maneuver was by standing before a full-length mirror, bending over, and peering between my legs to see the wound. I'd gingerly remove the soiled gauze, clean myself, and insert another piece. It was gross; it was stinky; it was anything but glamorous.

About six weeks into this routine, with little improvement in the wound, I was caught by surprise by the red, upside-down face of the woman who looked back at me in the mirror. Her hair was spiked from the pull of gravity, and her eyes were blue and eager. Her commitment to me was firm: she was working hard to get me well, and she was determined to do whatever was necessary to heal. She stuffed the turkey devotedly and lovingly. She was no longer disgusted by it. She was gentle. She was kind. She was my best advocate. She was Me.

"I love you," I heard her say. Her face was flushed red from hanging upside down. She smiled at me from between my legs. I stood upright, looked in the mirror, and for the first time in many months, I was no longer in battle.

Somehow, I had accepted the situation. I had surrendered the fight, the anger, the resistance, and I was doing whatever was necessary without resentment. There was no self-blame, no self-reproach. There was, however, anticipation, intense bouts of fear, and days of sadness. The wound wasn't healing, and that was seriously problematic. But together, the woman in the mirror and I would keep going, keep moving on. We had an abundance of love and support. Somehow we would make it through. All of me knew that.

When I realized that the love I was fostering in myself was at the core of how I was enduring all this, I decided it was time to get back to my spiritual life. I had pretty much abandoned it after my first diagnosis, because I couldn't square that we create our own reality or that we are cocreators with God. I hadn't been able to accept that whatever happens is an opportunity to grow. After my first diagnosis and the suffering I had experienced with the treatment, my spiritual views had gone out the window. Now it was time to reopen the window and let the fresh air of hope and peace fill my mind.

I've never been a Bible reader, but I've had a long and powerful thirst to know and communicate with God. I love that we live in a time of so many great spiritual teachers.

I devoured the work of Eckhart Tolle to learn to be present. Byron Katie taught me how to reframe my story so that it didn't hurt so much. I listened every night to Deepak Chopra's audiobook *The Soul of Healing Meditations.* Buddhist masters such as Thich Nhat Hahn and Pema Chödrön comforted me with an understanding of the ubiquity of love. I read Wayne Dyer and Marianne Williamson for inspiration. Jerry and Esther Hicks gave me all I needed in order to feel more empowered and stay focused on what I wanted. I longed to find meaning in my experience, so I turned to Viktor Frankl.

I also began to toy with the idea that maybe, just maybe, my cancer was related to my emotional self. I committed to cleaning out my emotional closets to see what I had been storing. Maybe I would learn something about myself, about why the cancer had returned.

In a visit with Dr. O., I told him I was going to do a thorough cleaning of my emotional self to see if there was anything there that might be contributing to the cancer.

He shrunk before my very eyes. "I hate when people do that," he said soberly.

"Do what?" I asked.

"Blame themselves for getting cancer."

"No, it's not about blame."

"You've already been through hell. Why would you want to blame yourself for it? Cancer has nothing to do with emotions or diet or anything. If you were a smoker, or obese, or any number of things, then we could talk. But you're in great shape. It's not fair to blame yourself. Promise me you won't do that."

"I promise."

I wanted to elaborate, but it was hard to articulate the difference between blaming yourself for what happens and taking responsibility. Blame indicates that something went seriously wrong and that you have failed. Blame suggests that you knew better but screwed up big time. Blame swims in guilt, which generates a destructive path of self-loathing.

Taking responsibility, on the other hand, begins by admitting that we don't have the answers; indeed, we know very little. But taking responsibility also consists of going on a journey of discovery. It accepts that there is a bigger story at play. It contends that this physical life is the vehicle through which we will discover what we currently don't know about the bigger part of ourselves. Perhaps we'll sense the higher design of our soul. Maybe we'll perceive how a past life has feathered into current circumstances. We may even stumble upon our life's purpose. Most of us tap into the God-given power that we all possess inside.

Taking responsibility means accepting that, for whatever reason, the situations we find ourselves in have meaning—meaning that can bring us closer to God, closer to knowing who we really are, and that can ultimately show us how to draw from the source of our own divine intelligence. Knowing this doesn't necessarily give order to chaos, but it does provide context and spiritual nourishment.

I began to see the cancer as *mine,* much like an arm or a leg. It was mine, and I began to attend to it not only physically, but also emotionally.

Meanwhile, the wound still wasn't healing. Dr. W. hospitalized me and scraped out the dead skin, hoping that new skin would surface. It didn't. He then put me on what's called a wound vac. It's a device that sucks out the old, wet skin, thus creating an opportunity for new skin to grow. After two attempts, however, I had the same severe allergic reaction to the tape that adhered the tubes to my body, so that was no longer an option.

Two months after my original surgery, the wound site was worse than ever. Desperation sank in.

"What do you want from me, God?" I hissed. "What do you want from me?! I'm doing everything I can fucking do! Why won't you let me heal?"

I punched the air, kicked my legs against the mattress, writhed with fury. Tika leapt from the bed. I threw myself on it, wept, and gave myself the only escape I knew—slumber.

Had I neglected to reinstate my spiritual life, I don't know how I would have made it through those next few weeks. Depressed and fearful that the doctors could do nothing for me, I lay in bed most days staring out the window, watching the sky, or reclining on the couch to distract myself with Turner Classic Movies.

Then Rita came to visit. She's an old friend from Telluride who, several years back, had escorted her husband to his death after he contracted AIDS. After Brian's death, Rita became a counselor. Her compassion, gentle wisdom, and playful humor were alluring, sweet, and comforting.

Rita sat in the chair next to my bed. We talked. She was no stranger to despair. She knew things were hard for me, and she felt my despair. Our conversation ceased. She smiled at me, and I smiled back at her. We looked into each other's eyes and held the gaze. She reached out and took my hand.

Without moving our eyes from each other, we were suddenly taken over by an awareness of a force much larger than ourselves, a force of immeasurable magnitude. It engulfed us. My body became light. The room was transformed. We stared into each other's eyes, which were flowing with tears. I felt a vibration of ubiquitous, all-encompassing love fill my body from head to toe. I believe it was a glimpse into the loving heart of God.

"There's nothing but love," Rita whispered, as though we were both on the verge of discovering a well-protected secret for the first time.

"I know," I agreed ecstatically.

The moment passed. We released hands and silently basked in the miracle. It was an experience we still speak of and one that I will never forget.

Not long after that, Susan, a beautiful, upbeat friend and public-health nurse called. "What can I do for you?" she asked. "Everyone is concerned about you, and we want to do something."

"I don't know. Maybe a massage. I want to do things like that, you know, like Reiki, acupuncture, healing touch. But insurance won't cover it, and we're broke. You could pay for a massage." I also wanted to resume my sessions with Bertrand.

Susan delivered more. She e-mailed friends and family all over the country, announcing that she was starting an alternative-healing fund. She helped me open a bank account devoted entirely to their donations. She wrote a letter informing people of where they could send the money. And she told them that the donations would be anonymous, so if people didn't want to give or couldn't, they wouldn't be embarrassed. The gratitude I felt toward Susan for that simple act of kindness lifted me for weeks.

After the rashes imposed by the wound vac cleared up, I visited Dr. W. again. Following our familiar and ever-so-intimate routine, I rolled to one side, opened the curtains of my butt, and waited for a comment. When he was finished with the exam, he stood and looked at the wall. In his absentminded-professor manner, he said nothing, just shifted his weight as he stared at the wall some more.

"I'm waiting," I said, now on my back.

"Oh, yeah, well...," he drifted off again. "Let me, let me...," he stumbled, and then sat and wheeled himself back over to me, Alice in tow, her white tennis shoes squeaking. I instinctively rolled to one side.

"I think...," he said.

Alice urged him on. "What do you see?"

"Let's, ah, there's something ... Alice, get me a speculum."

"What?" I cried. "Why a speculum?"

"Oh, I think there's ... I can see a little rent in there."

Rent, to me, is what you pay to stay in someone else's house. Alice saw the look on my face. "What he means is a tear in the skin," she explained.

"Where's the tear?"

"I just ... I don't ... let me ... lay on your back," he directed in his halting way.

I did. He placed the speculum inside me without any lubricant. I yelped. Alice quickly found some petroleum jelly. He lubed up the metal and inserted it again. Pain shot through me and didn't go away.

Then something strange happened. A rapid collage of images—ten, twenty, thirty?—passed before me. They were images of women throughout history being sexually abused or mutilated. I felt like I was transported through time, feeling their pain, carrying their pain. I tried to stifle the tears, but they lurched from me like the screams of the women in my head. Eddie squeezed my hand.

Dr. W. was awkwardly and sincerely apologetic. He was right, though; there was a tiny tear in the skin between my rectum and vagina.

"How did that get there?" I whined, still shaking off the images in my mind.

"I don't know," he replied. "Maybe when they did the surgery. But it needs to be fixed if you ever want to have sex again."

Eddie and I looked at each other longingly. "That would be good," my husband said whimsically.

Dr. W. considered the situation and came up with yet another plan. Between the rent in the tissue and the fact that the wound wasn't healing, he thought that the best thing we could do was a skin flap.

A familiar term. The thing that the surgeon in Denver decided was unnecessary. Surgery. Again.

In my pedestrian way, I thought a skin flap meant taking a piece of skin from my thigh and sewing shut the opening of the wound, creating a literal flap that would close it up. The procedure is far more dramatic than that. They remove the gracilis muscle from a leg and insert it into the wound, which offers a fresh, new batch of blood supply to the site. The gracilis muscle isn't a small muscle; it runs from the knee to the groin on the inside of the leg. It's long, thin, and, apparently, unnecessary, or at least you can function just fine without it. Dr. W. assured me that once I healed, I wouldn't miss it. Given his sense of humor, I wasn't sure if he was kidding or telling the truth.

Removing an entire muscle was frightening. I imagined myself gimping around, my colostomy bag flapping in the wind. What a sight.

***

I had the surgery on November 18, 2007, but each day that Dr. W. came to check on me, instead of hearing good news, I would hear the snipping of his scissors.

"What are you cutting?" I asked. I felt nothing.

Dr. W. didn't answer. Robin said at last, "It's dead skin."

"What dead skin?"

Quiet again.

"What dead skin? What are you cutting?" I demanded.

Finally Robin answered. "The skin that is supposed to be healing to close up the wound isn't doing well. He's cutting that dead skin away."

It wasn't healing—not the day after surgery, not a week after surgery. I fell into a deep depression. Dr. W. tried to help by ordering a special bed for me that promised greater comfort. By then, however, I was practically inconsolable.

It was Thanksgiving. My family and some dear friends came to my hospital room, covered a drab table with a bright cloth, brought out turkey and all the fixings, and drank wine from paper cups. I ate little. They toasted to my health, but I held no hope for recovery. I felt nothing but disdain for everyone and everything. I was locked up tight, seething with gloom, and wanted nothing more than to crawl into a hole and disappear forever.

At the end of the meal, Lyric asked if she could spend the night with me. Eddie beckoned a friendly nurse, who agreed that it was fine, even though it was against the rules, and she brought pillows and blankets for a large reclining chair.

As I watched my beautiful young daughter drift to sleep, my heart slowly softened and then opened. The innocence and wonder of that single, most beautiful creature—my daughter, a perfectly imperfect human being for whom I possessed more love than I could comprehend—and the sight of her asleep in a chair, resuscitated me. And once again I accepted that there was something in this experience for me to discover. I was on the ride of my life, and even though it was hard, I would make it to the finish line. I would.

Three days later, Dr. W. announced that the gracilis muscle was finally taking to the skin inside of the wound. It was healing. Soon I would be home.

Generous donations were pouring into the alternative-healing fund. I began regular treatments of acupuncture, chiropractic, healing touch, and massage, as well as having sessions with Bertrand. Not a week went by without me being the grateful recipient of the generosity bestowed upon me by my friends and family.

One day, serendipitously, I received a letter from my closest friend on the West Coast and a card from my closest friend on the East Coast. Both contained liberal checks that would enable me to buy a microcurrent machine, a medical device that would help expedite healing. It had only been a few days since I asked God to help me find a way to buy the $2,000 apparatus. Upon opening their cards, the exact amount necessary to purchase the machine sat on my lap. I wept with gratitude.

I was beginning to perceive the abundance and overwhelming magnanimity of the universe. I started to focus on what I was grateful for, rather than on what I didn't have. I still couldn't sit upright, but I could drive if I leaned forward and to one side. Who cares if I looked like Cruella de Vil. I couldn't bathe, but I could shower. I couldn't exercise, but I could walk to the mailbox. I couldn't replace the ugly tiles in my kitchen, but I could peer out my living room window and watch the red towering rocks of the Colorado National Monument flirt with the light of a boastful sun.

The months that it took to recover afforded me time and motivation to explore my inner, emotional landscape. I trusted that there must be an emotional element to getting cancer—especially a second time. So unlike what I did after my first diagnosis, this time I pursued whatever thread I could follow to a grievance held deep within or a dormant upset that remained unresolved. I found plenty to work on, including judgments I had harbored toward family members and, of course, myself.

Bing, my stunningly intuitive acupuncturist, busted me every time I slipped into self-pity. He coached me on how to become empowered through forgiveness, focusing on what I wanted, taking ownership of my life, and believing in wellness.

After months of reading books by spiritual teachers and delving inside myself, I realized that to be free of the fears, anxieties, and judgments I'd carried for a lifetime, I would have to change the paradigm of my thoughts and responses to life. I drew from my own experience and came up with the five dominant qualities I believed were essential for healing and wholeness: acceptance, surrender, gratitude, forgiveness, and love.

I gladly worked hard to live out these qualities. In the course of my spiritual studies, I was startled to see how deeply fear had been programmed into me and had followed me throughout my entire life. I was always waiting for the other shoe to drop. I had major, albeit very discreet, issues with trust—trusting myself, trusting God, trusting Life. I carried tension that I had worn for so long, and it wasn't until I took it off that I could feel how heavy it had been—and how normal I'd thought it was. In my journey toward wholeness, my life was changing dramatically for the better. I fully grasped that it was due to the cancer that I had grown into a woman I much preferred to hang out with. I was literally in awe of and more in love with life than ever before, more alive than ever before. The freedom that cleaning out my emotional closets provided was worth every moment of the labor necessary to discard what no longer served me.

In May 2008, the wound finally closed up completely. It took nine months of Betsy's care and working with Dr. W., but finally the skin came together. Dr. W. gave me a warm embrace and announced that he had never been so happy to release a patient from his care.

Episode 3: Spiritual

In August of 2008, exactly two years after my first diagnosis and one year after the second, a routine CT scan revealed a small mass located next to my sciatic nerve.

"It's probably nothing," Dr. R. said sweetly. "We can wait three months and see if it grows, but if I were you, I'd want to know now."

I put my head down on his desk and sat perfectly still. No tears. No emotion at all. I didn't need a biopsy to confirm it; I knew what it was.

A week later, it was confirmed. This time, they called it metastasized.

That's when the tears came uncontrollably. I had been through so much—done so much to heal—and now this. Dr. R. had little to offer.

"I'm pretty sure we can take care of the tumor that's there. But it's what's to come that ... it's what's to come...," he said in a near whisper.

Ed and I spent two weeks, mostly in the privacy of our bedroom, trying to keep the measure of our terror from impacting the kids. I would collapse into tears on the bed, he'd hold me, and together we'd ask *why*—after we'd been through so much and with such a good prognosis—why was this happening?

I tried to make sense of my situation, yet it all kept coming up meaningless. Still, I had learned by then that it was up to me to find meaning in the situation and to do something with it. I had already decided that I would not cave in to the gloom and doom and do nothing. I'd learn about eating raw foods and work with alternative healers. I simply would not fold into the expectation of a bad statistic.

Ed and I agreed that if the cancer was in my system, I had better fill my system with the very best possible nutrients. I rifled through Kris Carr's book *Crazy Sexy Cancer Tips.* At the age of twenty-seven, Kris had been diagnosed with twenty-four inoperable and incurable cancerous tumors on her liver. In her book, she writes that everything came together for her after she went to the Living Foods Institute (LFI) in Atlanta.[2]

I booked myself at the Institute for a twelve-day rendezvous with how to prepare and live on raw foods. I also decided that I would start working with Dr. Barre Lando, DC, MICP, a brilliant alternative doctor who employed an eclectic and cutting-edge protocol. I called him early one morning while the kids were asleep. I sat shaking as we talked.

"First, there is no such thing as disease," he said. "There are conditions that occur, and people put labels on them, then expect these conditions to act the way they did for every other person given that label. These people don't consider that it's just a set of conditions, and those conditions can change. It's all about learning who you really are. You have the power," he said, "to reverse the conditions right now. But you have to believe that."

I didn't.

He then launched into the research he'd done and how he'd put his scientifically based programs together, supported by samples of blood, urine, and saliva. The idea that there was no such thing as disease was a strong statement that took time to absorb, but I wanted to believe in his protocol. Then he said, "You can either engage in war on your body, which you've already done twice now, or you can engage in peace. Peace is my approach."

He reported that he had seen people completely heal from cancer. He assured me that not only was it possible to heal, but also that by working *with* the body instead of *against* it (in other words, "burning and poisoning"), the chances of lasting recovery were greater.

"There's no guarantee this approach will work for you," he cautioned. "No one can give you a guarantee; it's just a matter of which way you want to go. The truth is, it doesn't really matter what treatment you choose. What matters is that you fully believe in whatever treatment you do. Ask yourself what's motivating you to choose the treatment you're going for. That will tell you a lot."

Fear was motivating me to go with whatever conventional treatment an oncologist could find. Hope was motivating me to work with this man and heal. Really heal. I vowed to see him as soon as I could make it out to California, where he lived.

Before I left for Atlanta, I visited Dr. R. again. He was upbeat because of a new type of radiation called CyberKnife, which he felt could handle the latest tumor. Essentially, CyberKnife is the next generation of radiation. Unlike the "wide field" radiation I'd had before, this entered the body at hundreds of different points, all of which received a very low dose of radiation. Consequently, the rays would not interfere with healthy tissue. When all the points converged at the tumor, their combined dose apparently obliterated the cancerous tissue. There were supposedly no side effects and no debilitating burns.

Dr. R. was hopeful about the technology. I was open, but unsure. I liked the idea of working out my health issues with radishes rather than radiation. Painful experience had proven that the big guns just hadn't worked for me before, so why would they this time? Dr. R. said it was my best option. He reiterated that the cancer had metastasized and there wasn't anything else he knew to do. His eyes were fixed on the cold linoleum floor. I told him I'd check it out, but I also wanted to share my other plans with him.

"Alternatives," he said in a soft voice, "won't help others. If you get on a clinical trial, it might help others in your same situation."

"But there's been a lot of success with this diet and other alternative ways of—"

"All that gives you is false hope," he interrupted.

False hope? What is false hope, anyway? Is it a term that people thrust upon treatments they don't understand? Or does it mean investing in something that ultimately doesn't pay off? If so, that's exactly what happened to me after undergoing chemo, radiation, and surgery! In my case, the scientific promise of a 90 percent cure rate is what hadn't paid off. *That* reeked of false hope.

"Alternative treatments," he reiterated, "give false hope. I'm dealing with reality."

I flashed back to something that had come to me while in the tunnel of an MRI machine: just as beauty is in the eye of the beholder, reality is in the mind of the believer. I nodded with a new and deep understanding. I was on an adventure that had taken me out of Dr. R.'s territory, and now Dr. R. and I occupied completely different realities.

I asked the next question purely out of curiosity, because I knew he was a religious man. "What about spontaneous remission? It happens."

"Well..." He took a moment and pondered. I could only imagine what might go on in the mind of a well-meaning doctor whose high-tech science had failed him and who, in med school, isn't taught how to talk about miracles. "I'm a man of science, but I'm also a man of God—and God can do whatever he wants."

"Right," I said. "I think so too."

We sat in silence. I had grown to love Dr. R. He had done everything he knew to rid me of cancer, but what he knew didn't work. After one too many beats of silence, we said an awkward good-bye.

A few days later, I was crippled with fear. What if Dr. R. was right? What if I was investing in hocus-pocus that would lead nowhere? What if there was nothing that anyone could do to help?

Motivated by the type of exhaustion that terror breeds, I decided to see a therapist. Diana's bright eyes and clear presence welcomed me into her office. "I'm afraid I might be dying," I told her and then explained the situation. She knew my history. She knew the physical agony and emotional suffering I had endured. She knew the fears that pushed against me. She knew me, and she also knew that I was *not* dying.

"Look at you!" she bellowed. "You're not dying! You have a centimeter-sized tumor in your butt! Other than that, you're perfectly healthy, and your doctor has no idea what's to come! This could be the last vestige of cancer within you! It could be all there is, and yet he's leading you to believe that you could be *dying?* This is outrageous!"

Her fervor was infectious. She was right. I wasn't dying! I was alive and healthy in every other respect. I was very much alive! I felt good! I had a small tumor, yes, but I absolutely was *not* dying.

Diana also told me about a book she was reading by Dr. Candace Pert entitled *Molecules of Emotion: The Science Behind Mind-Body Medicine*.[3] The book describes how our emotions can impact our cells.

"You've gotta read it," she beamed. "You'll understand what your choices are. And you *do* have choices."

I told her I was thinking about writing a book. She smiled again, nodding silently. Embracing me, she said, "Yes. You have a book to write. You have choices, and you are not dying."

This much was absolutely certain; I had no symptoms, and I was in no pain. Diana's perspective and the conditions of my situation had given me the cosmic nod to move forward in a way that I was determined would heal me completely—on every level and in every way. I walked out of Diana's office with confidence for the first time since my last visit with Dr. R.

Bouncing off the premise in Dr. Pert's book, I accepted that the cancer must have something to do with the energetic tone set within me. Even Einstein said that we're made up of nothing but energy. I had already done great work on forgiveness and releasing old fears and grievances, but I knew there must be more work to do.

So began weeks of contemplating the puzzle of why the cancer returned. In her book *Intuitive Wellness: Using Your Body's Inner Wisdom to Healing*, Laura Alden Kamm describes cancer cells as "fiercely independent and rebellious." She writes that the core emotional issues usually relate to fear, deep sadness, and grief, and that the spiritual intelligence of rogue cells are rooted in being afraid and restricted in life, a perception of being cut off from love or unable to truly express one's uniqueness.[4]

I reviewed my life and soon focused on the time when Eddie and I had come within inches of splitting up. During that time, there had been more conflict than I'd thought I could stomach, and I had often found myself physically stricken with anguish, fearful that we wouldn't make it as a couple, and equally terrified that we'd stay together, but remain miserable. I felt stuck and angry. I was absolutely experiencing fear, deep sadness, and grief over what I perceived as the loss of a good marriage. These were the very emotions that described the energetic nature behind cancer cells, according to Kamm.

Thankfully, we had made it through those difficult years. To this day, I maintain that the intense negative emotions I felt and the years I cast blame against Eddie were part of what broke down the cells in my body, creating an environment for cancer to thrive.

Kamm's insights graced me with another significant revelation. One day while driving alone in the car, I asked myself, "What part of myself have I left behind so there has to be rebellion?"

In a furious flash, an image came to my mind's eye. A tall, lean, teenaged girl with long blonde hair appeared before me in a rage. "You abandoned me!" she screamed. "You left me behind, and I hate you for it!"

She didn't resemble me, but there was no doubt that she was me. I knew instantaneously that she was my creative self.

Since young adulthood, I had dreamed of being a successful writer. As an adult, playwriting was what attracted me most. The choices I made to marry, have children, and move to a small town in western Colorado catapulted me away from my dreams. Throughout the years, the demands of a life I had willingly chosen slowly chipped away at my creative ambitions, and I was haunted by that lost dream.

I didn't know how to reconcile the angst within me. My passion for writing was the very stuff that had lit me up in high school. It's what had driven me in college, where my first play was produced. It had given me the strength and confidence to move—by myself—to Hollywood and take a stab at the entertainment business. My creative heat was also what attracted Ed to me and me to him. He is made up of the same fire. In fact, when I first met Ed, he'd been writing scripts and working as a still photographer on movie sets to pay the bills. He was—and still is—a soulful, talented musician. We met, married, and had kids. The rest is history.

I didn't abandon my dreams entirely, however. Every year, I enjoyed productions of my plays in small theatres across the country. Still, those remote successes weren't even close to what I had dreamed. But with a mortgage to pay, a job to keep, a marriage in need, and children to raise, that's just the way it was. I had resigned myself to a life that was good in many ways, but one that left me feeling, in a very deep and private place, that I had betrayed myself.

I was startled by the rage of the blonde girl in my mind's eye—and the fact that she was at least partially right. I hadn't wanted to be a starving artist. I had wanted the comforts of a nice home, a functional car, and I especially craved a loving union with a man and children. I had chosen those things willingly.

"I didn't totally neglect you," I protested. "I've written plays and done creative things for years. Plus I was never going to give up a family for writing. I wanted that just as much."

"But you came into this life to create, and now you're working a job that has nothing to do with me and giving the rest of your time to your kids. You left me behind!"

She crossed her arms and turned her back to me. I couldn't argue with her. In another quick flash, her name came to me: Raven.

"Raven?" I asked aloud, laughing uncomfortably at the character who had appeared in the confidential world of my mind. "How can your name be Raven? You don't even have black hair."

I was just about to turn on to the freeway when two large black crows flew in front of my windshield nearly smashing it. By the time I slammed on the brakes, they were gone. Never before or since have I come so close to hitting birds while driving.

"OK," I said shaking with excitement as much as with adrenaline. "Your name is Raven."

Still, her back was to me, just as mine had been to her—my dreams—for years. Although I did what I could in the context of my life, I was ignoring the very calling I had felt since childhood. There were times when I felt sick with sadness because I wasn't living out that part of myself. It was just as Kamm's book said: I had been grieving the loss of this part of myself for years; I hadn't been expressing my creative uniqueness. I completely understood Raven's defiance and anger.

Her expectations had been strong, and I had failed her. Her image vanished, but at least I had a handle on what I was up against. Or, more pointedly, what part of me was so deeply against me.

***

My journey was well underway by the time I saw an oncology specialist in Denver. I told him I didn't want to hear his prognosis; I only wanted his ideas on solutions. He looked slightly perplexed and then explained CyberKnife, the radiation that Dr. R. thought was my best shot. My mind was wide open to whatever could help me. Working with Dr. Lando in California, eating raw foods, and undergoing CyberKnife were all showing up as compatible. They were a combination I could live with, believe in, and fully embrace.

A week later, I attended a five-day workshop at the Shambhala Mountain Center outside of Fort Collins, Colorado. It was called "Healthy Body, Happy Mind" and was facilitated by Dr. Mark Hyman. I had signed up for it prior to my last diagnosis, and I was considering canceling, as I was still in shock. Yet I had a strong feeling that it would be good for me to go.

It was the right decision. On the first day of the workshop, Dr. Hyman said, "There's no such thing as disease." I laughed out loud. So Dr. Lando wasn't the only one who proposed this radical notion. I took this as a very good omen.

The conference was about Dr. Hyman's belief that physical disturbances, caused either by food allergies or vitamin or mineral deficiencies, are behind emotional issues such as bipolar disorder, borderline personality, and manic depression. His ideas fed directly into my belief in the relationship between the mind and the body and how they are constantly at play.

At the close of one session, I approached Dr. Hyman. "How powerful do you think the mind really is?" I asked. "Can it heal us?"

"This is the most powerful pharmacy in the universe," he said, tapping on his temple. "Right here."

That was all I needed.

***

Meditation and prayer became an even bigger part of my life. Raven often came to me during meditations, and I willingly listened to her and engaged in silent conversation. About a month after she first came to me, and following many candid and often painful dialogues, she appeared in the space I allowed for her in my mind. She sat on a folding chair and watched me, saying nothing. She no longer looked angry. She seemed more relaxed than I'd ever seen before. I reached out my hand and asked if she wanted to meditate with me. She gave a hint of a smile, nodded, and walked over to me. Then, like in an old sixties movie, she blended into me, and we became one. That was the end of our separation. She had forgiven me.

Today, she is quiet and content. Each time I see a crow, raven, or any black bird, we smile.

***

By the time I attended the Living Foods Institute in Atlanta, I was prepared to leave old habits behind. I happily traded in hamburgers for jicama and processed foods for living foods. That was what I could do for my body, but my mind also needed a new path, one that would allow me to really and truly believe I would heal.

Days are long at the LFI. Each morning, we learned to prepare a feast of delicious raw meals. We spent most afternoons addressing toxic emotional issues and how they feed into our bodies. I had already done much of the work they proposed, but I was happy to review it. My two weeks there were intense, joyful, and also often filled with fear. I was scheduled to undergo CyberKnife when I returned home, but the more time I spent in Atlanta, the less certain I became that I wanted to subject myself to more radiation. The doctor had told me that if the tumor grew and attached itself to the sciatic nerve, they wouldn't be able to do the procedure because there was a risk of destroying the nerve, leaving me with a useless leg. Even so, I wasn't sure.

One day, about midway through the conference, I was paralyzed with fear once again. I didn't know if the path I was choosing was right or would work. I didn't know if doing CyberKnife would hurt more than help. I was afraid of dying. A menacing gang of doubts knocked me down and towered over me. They insisted that this raw food thing was stupid, that tracking and releasing emotional aspects was horseshit. They mocked me and said the cancer was just the product of another random act in a senseless universe, and that nothing I would do was going to work.

I resisted the doubts, but they hovered over me. I felt the weight and fate of my life upon me, and I didn't have the strength to endure them. I didn't have the skill. The truth was, I wasn't trusting the path that I had chosen.

During a break, I walked to a nearby park, masking my tears from passersby. I had never before experienced that kind of fear. I had been so sure that eating raw foods would help. All my alternative docs said it was a great idea. Brenda Cobb, the owner of LFI, cured herself of cancer by eating raw. So did the woman with the brain tumors. But those doubts, those thugs, were kicking at my conviction, laughing at my foolishness.

I came upon a bench and sat. I knew this gang well, and I needed to send them walking or I might be converted. The only thing I knew to do was pray. I closed my eyes.

"OK, God." I whispered, tears pooling at my chin. "Help me. Please help me."

In a moment, it became clear: I didn't have to do this by myself. It wasn't all up to me. I had support—not only from Eddie, Mom, and all the people who loved me, but also from God, spirits, angels, and a universe of nonphysical beings.

I opened my eyes and peered out at the vast park before me. There, almost as though I could touch them and as far as I could see, were translucent white outlines of ethereal bodies. Most were standing and cheering. Others swung gleefully from tree limbs. Some lined the horizon, clapping. A few did cartwheels; others stood on their heads.

The huge audience of these nonphysical beings stretched on forever. Every direction I turned, they were there, standing and clapping, dancing, throwing their arms up with joy, squatting in trees, or swinging from branches. They were there for me. All of them.

"You are supported," I heard them say. "And you are loved."

At that moment, I let go of having to heal myself by myself.

"OK, God," I whispered again, wiping away the tears. "I'll clean up my diet and my thoughts. The rest is up to you. Thank you."

The relief was huge. The gang of doubts vanished. I walked back to the

Institute and made guacamole with the rest of my new tribe.

***

After my first two diagnoses, I had welcomed the love, participation, and contribution of friends and family—even strangers. This time around, however, I felt the need for strict privacy. I had to protect myself from other people's fears about what a third diagnosis might mean and their doubts about how I was choosing to heal. I shared the news only with my immediate family, my closest in-town friends, and my office mates. By then, Robin, the ostomy nurse, had become a treasured friend. Her spiritual philosophy fed me daily nourishment.

I felt strange about withholding the news from dear and devoted friends, those who had so vigorously and lovingly supported me in the past. But I needed every ounce of energy to invest in myself. I couldn't carry anyone else's skepticism because every now and then I had too much of my own. It was an intensely delicate and internal time.

To support myself, I wanted to hear about how other people had healed. I needed to know both how they did it and that they had succeeded. I needed to hear their stories to help me create my own.

I was eating raw foods and feeling better than I had ever felt before. I was sharpening my mind with an understanding of its power, and I still wasn't sure I wanted to do the CyberKnife. Dr. C., who offered the procedure, was very respectful and said that he understood.

"But don't you think it's best to do everything you possibly can?" he asked in a gentle, noninvasive manner.

I did, but I was also dubious. And I knew that I would need to find a way to believe in it for the procedure to work most effectively. By then, Dr. Bruce Lipton's book *The Biology of Belief: Unleashing the Power of Consciousness, Matter, and Miracles* had taught me about the enormous power of the subconscious mind and how it can sabotage even our strongest conscious desires.[5] I decided to visit a hypnotherapist to try and access the resistance toward the CyberKnife that was hidden behind the shade of my conscious mind. After only one session, I was fully onboard with doing the CyberKnife.

The treatments lasted only five days. I spent my evenings in a hotel in Boulder as Barack Obama won the presidential election. I was full of hope for my country and for myself. I returned home with only minor side effects and a bag full of seeds that I intended to sprout for my new culinary regimen.

***

I was done with conventional treatment, but my quest for wholeness continued. I poured through books about self-healing. I read daily from Dr. David Hawkins' book, *Healing and Recovery.* Myrtle Fillmore, cofounder of the Unity Church, hugely influenced me through her book *How to Let God Help You.* Filmore had healed herself from terminal tuberculosis in the mid 1800s, and her philosophy can be reduced to a single line from the book: "The body and its functions respond readily and fully to the bidding of the mind. So you see, healing is always assured!"[6] After reading her book, I began a dialogue with my cells and practiced healing visualization every night.

I committed myself to the philosophy of Abraham, as channeled through Esther Hicks, and paid full attention to being well rather than having cancer. Of course, I would slip up and be gripped with terror that I was wrong, that emotions and mental focus had nothing to do with cancer, and that I was doomed. But then, I would circle back to my highest, deepest, broadest intention, which was to heal fully.

I flew out to California and met with Dr. Lando, who put me on a strict regimen of herbs and homeopathic remedies.

***

My life changed dramatically during those months. I became acutely aware of a power within that I had never needed to tap into before. I was lifted in spirit and lightened in load. The food I ate was pure and good; the thoughts I had were positive; the gratitude I felt was tremendous. I found happiness in the depths of myself.

In February I had my first follow-up scan with Dr. C. The tumor had not grown, and that was good news.

"But it's still there?" I asked, surprised.

"Yes, but it hasn't grown. That's what we want," the nurse reported.

"I'll take care of it," I said, smiling.

"What?"

"I'll take care of the tumor."

"OK," she said, unsure of how to respond. "But this is good news."

As happy as I was, the months that followed were full of losses. In March my mother's cousin, whom I was close with, died of pancreatic cancer. Then Herbert, who'd brought me baggy pants after surgery, was hospitalized with complications in his heart. Finally, in May, after months of vaginal bleeding, my mother was diagnosed with very aggressive acute myeloid leukemia (AML). The type of chemo it required would kill her. She was given eight weeks to live.

I spent hours looking for alternative solutions for my mother. I contacted several of the doctors whom I had interviewed for this book, but the people I spoke to had not successfully treated AML.

Mom went to Denver, and with my sister Lynn, she met with a variety of specialists. One doctor said there was a chemo that would work, but Medicare didn't cover it. It would cost tens of thousands of dollars and alter her quality of life exponentially. My mother was a lively seventy-nine-year-old with few financial reserves. It was all overwhelming.

She returned from her trip clear about three things: she would spend the summer in Estes Park with her sisters, she would take my family and me to Hawaii in the fall, and then she would find the money and do the chemo.

The next day she had another stroke, her third. This time it was significant, and she would not be able to return to the life she had lived before. This time I could take care of her: I gently took away her car keys, quickly found an assisted-living home, and immediately moved her essential items into it.

The stroke had impacted her speech, her logic, and her balance. Still, she recovered remarkably well, and three weeks later I drove her to Estes Park. We had a wonderful drive over the Continental Divide, laughing and talking about her life. I knew it would be our last trip "over the hill" to our longtime family gathering place in Estes Park. I held her hand, and we yammered on, avoiding the topic that gave us no choices and little time.

Seven days later, I held her hand once again as she died.

My mother's life had not been easy. There were strong indications that her stepfather had sexually abused her when she was a young girl. As an adult, her relationships with men were terribly dysfunctional. She went through four marriages and, after feeling victimized in one way or another, terminated each one. Six months before she died, she told me she thought penises were weapons.

Mom was a deeply wounded person who never learned to love herself. I found it poignant and relevant that her cancer first manifested through vaginal bleeding, the place that she had surely been violated as a child and throughout her youth—the place where her wounds had never healed.

As I watched my sweet mother gasp her last breaths, I prayed that she would finally find peace, finally become whole, finally heal all that she could not face or admit in this life, and finally be free.

As I sat with her in the gold light of that ending day, just before my sisters and children were to arrive, I was struck by how you cannot save anyone else—no one, no matter how much you love them. You can only save yourself—or die trying.

I was also struck by how natural death is. It didn't frighten me. It was the course of things. In her case, it was the only course left.

The tree my mother planted for me stands tall and healthy in her backyard. She never placed a plaque beneath it with my name etched on it. For that, I am grateful.

Both Farrah Fawcett and our dear friend Herbert died that same week. Then, to top it off, my dog Gradie got cancer on her foot. One year after getting a toe removed, Gradie sits beside me now, anxious to go on a walk. Tika's tail continues to wag.

During the flurry of my aunt's death and the storm of Mom's diagnosis and death, I didn't have any follow-up scans until July, a year after my third diagnosis. When the time finally came, I was once again frozen with fear. What if my approach had been wrong? What if I were riddled with cancer? What if the malicious gang of doubts had been right?

The scan was conducted in Grand Junction and digitally sent to Dr. C. in Boulder. Eddie and I paced the house, awaiting his call.

When the phone rang, the nurse from Dr. C.'s office was out of breath. "We have verrrry goooood news," she bellowed. "It's gone. It has vanished! The tumor vanished! Your cancer is resolved!"

We jumped like cheerleaders, and Eddie swept me into his arms. We cried and held each other so tightly you'd have thought we were one.

The journey isn't over—as long as I live, it will continue—but the path I had chosen proved worthy of pursuit. I felt myself relax in a way that I hadn't been able to until I got the news that the cancer was resolved. That's truly what I had done to heal—resolved.

I resolved to continually weed out negative thinking and work through emotions that were prickly with anger, blame, resentment, and what I've come to know as toxic. I still do.

I resolved to put good food into my body and be aware of what my body needs, wants, doesn't tolerate, and on occasion must indulge in. I still do.

I resolved to exercise and be active, but to be gentle and have fun along the way. I still do.

I resolved to be true to my purpose and create clear intentions with every new layer of life that reveals itself to me. I still do.

I resolved to be well. I still do.

The tears of joy I tasted the day I found out that my cancer was resolved were different than the ones born of sorrow, grief, and loss. They were sweet. They were mellow. They were soft. They still are.

For this is the great error of our day that the physicians separate the soul from the body.

HIPPOCRATES

CHAPTER 2

Forgiveness

Don't carry a grudge. While you're carrying a grudge, the other guy's out dancing.
BUDDY HACKETT

The act of forgiveness is perhaps the most powerful medicine we possess. It's also the most elusive. When we feel hurt, betrayed, deceived, abandoned, abused, dismissed, or disrespected to any degree, our immediate response is to fight or flee. Fighting is associated with courage, while fleeing suggests protecting ourselves. Forgiveness requires that we surpass the instinct to fight and redefine the meaning of self-preservation.

To rise above the understandable reaction to fight or flee, we are charged with making a deliberate choice. Ordinarily, we don't exercise that choice. Instead, we tend to *want* to duke it out, to dominate, to win; or maybe we *want* to walk away enraged or victimized in order to justify and fuel the anger and resentment we wear like armor.

Being treated badly, regardless of how slightly or severely, insults the native and correct understanding that we are absolutely worthy of being treated with respect, kindness, and love. That we should be honored is inborn knowledge. When we are not, the ego goes wild and tends to engage with glee in the blame game.

Cancer gives us plenty of reasons to feel angry and victimized. It may be the diagnosis itself, the painful and debilitating treatment, or the loss of our normal lives. We may also feel hurt and outrage at the expectation, imposed upon us by others, that we will die.

Then there are the frustrations of dealing with the current medical system, complete with insurance companies that double bill us or numb hospital bureaucrats who charge such exorbitant prices that we end up having to sell the ranch. Regardless, the cancer industry has forged a nearly nonnegotiable road for those who get diagnosed.

If those feelings of anger, resentment, victimization, and powerlessness somehow contributed to the creation of the disease, now is the time to dig down deep and begin the process of releasing. Chances are good that we didn't experience these feelings for the first time just after the diagnosis; these are probably old and familiar members of our inner emotional tribe.

To heal, truly and deeply, we are charged with somehow, in some way, bypassing the urge to retaliate, to cast blame, or to further ignite the justifications for remaining a victim. We must find the still and certain center of our hearts, the place that wants to release the grievances and find peace. It's the deepest part of our heart that knows, without doubt, that we are divine and there is no need to fight or blame. When we feel a tug to be still rather than to fight or flee, then we're closer to that center, a territory so subtle and sublime that it can easily be overlooked.

Giving up the battle is a hard concept in a culture that thrives on drama and adversity. Before I grasped this concept, I judged a friend whom I saw backing off from an argument with a coworker, a situation where my friend was clearly in the right and the coworker clearly in the wrong. I inquired why she was submitting, and she said, "I asked myself if I'd rather be *right* or at peace. I'd rather be at peace, so I'm letting it go." The ferocity in her eyes showed that this wasn't the easiest choice, but it was the best one. Plus, she was telling me in no uncertain terms that this was none of my business.

Each of us is responsible for finding the sweet spot where forgiveness dwells. Each of us is in charge of how deeply we let our upsets, anger, resentments, and sorrows run. We have the choice—always—to let those heavy emotions go. Forgiveness is the way.

It is essential to enact forgiveness with every grudge or judgment that surfaces, because in order to truly heal, we must admit once and for all that we are not victims. Rather, at our core, we are powerful, pure, loving, blissful, peaceful beings. Playing the victim keeps us bound to the laws of the ego. When we forgive, we sanction who we really are. We no longer need or want to be the victim, because forgiveness takes us beyond the rigid dictates of right and wrong. It delivers us to compassion and the acceptance that we occupy a complex world in which every point of view can be understood.

How do we do it? After all, we live in a relentless atmosphere of anger, fear, blame, revenge, outrage, and simplistic black-or-white, wrong-or-right dogmas. Radio and television talk-show hosts scream at us to be mad as hell and blame the "other" for the state of our ailing world. Forgiveness isn't a topic of discussion unless it's couched in sarcasm or cynicism. We cannot watch the news or look to media icons to learn the ways of forgiveness.

Do we dare look to preachers, priests, rabbis, and ministers to learn how to forgive? Only if we're lucky enough to find a church, a synagogue, or a mosque that's free of harsh opinions about those who practice life or faith in ways different from our own. Remarkably, judgment seems to be the backbone of many religions today, since political viewpoints have penetrated the pulpit and embroider scripture with partisan design.

There's nothing you and I can do about that. The machine is too big. We can, however, congregate at the cornerstones of our consciousness and weed out the judgments we possess and protect. Many of those judgments will feel deeply entrenched, leftover from childhood. Some will feel ancient, having followed us into this life from another. Others will be rooted in the current conclusions we have made. How or why our judgments and grievances exist doesn't ultimately matter. What does matter is letting them go.

Deciding to forgive is the first step. Whether we harbor a lifetime of anger or have just gotten caught up in a specific period of time or a particular incident, we must consciously and deliberately choose forgiveness.

After my second diagnosis, when I began taking responsibility for my cancer, I sat with a pad and pen and wrote down the names of every person who was important to me, followed by what I wanted to forgive them for and why I believed they did what they did. It went something like this:

Mom, I forgive you for never claiming your power and allowing people to walk all over you. I know you felt unworthy of intimacy and love, and this was one way of proving to yourself that you were right.

Dad, I forgive you for being sarcastic and critical. I know you did this because you felt powerless, and it was a way for you to feel more powerful or even superior. I also forgive you for being an alcoholic. I know you were verbally abused as a child, and you were so deeply wounded and sensitive that you drank to numb the pain.

For my stepfather, I wrote: *Stan, I forgive you for being angry, controlling, and meanspirited at times. I know you felt little control in your own life and that you were compelled to try to control others as a means of survival. I know you were intensely angry because you probably didn't get the kind of love you deserved as a child.*

And so on.

Sometimes after writing, I felt the forgiveness immediately. Other times, I simply planted the seed. Setting the intention to forgive through exercises like this will actually open the door for the act of forgiveness to find completion. I was astonished at how much lighter I felt after the exercises. Indeed, by releasing the negative convictions, anger, fear, resentment, and hurt—all very heavy emotions—I lifted a burden, and I felt freer and lighter. This was further evidence that carrying grievances hurt no one but myself.

It's not my place to judge others. But judgments do keep arising, and it's up to me to discharge them. If instead of passing through me, negative judgments take up residence within me, I proactively do what's necessary to release them. If exercises like what I just described don't work, I pray for help, because in the long run, *nothing* is more lethal to my body than being a cauldron for resentment and other heavy emotions. It may feel good for a moment to carry anger and cast blame, but over time it's deeply destructive. I learned that the hard way.

Freeing ourselves of poisonous emotions isn't just about forgiving the "other." Very often—indeed, more often than not—it's about forgiving ourselves.

Forgiving ourselves can be a difficult concept to grasp. We aren't taught that the worst abuse and neglect often comes from within, yet upon paying closer attention, it doesn't take us long to become aware of some intensely negative self-talk. Eventually, it becomes necessary to forgive ourselves for self-destructive behaviors, such as dishonoring ourselves by not speaking up or allowing our voices to be heard, by losing someone or something we loved because of neglect or lack of consideration, or by neglecting our bodies or life's purpose by giving into harmful addictions. We're masters at putting ourselves down.

Then there are all the ways in which we breed a negative environment by putting others down. This could include cutting comments we make about or to someone else, simple but wicked gossip, or our unspoken but toxic judgments—from criticizing the texture of someone's hair to dismissing them due to their gender. We're also masters at putting others down.

To reiterate, treating others or ourselves badly, regardless of how slightly or severely, insults the truth that we, and everyone else, are absolutely worthy of being treated with respect, kindness, and love. We have an inborn knowledge that we should honor all others and ourselves. When we do not, the ego goes wild and pummels us with guilt and blame for being a bad and worthless person, which only perpetuates the cycle of wanting to blame others so that we can feel better about ourselves.

We're all members of the gang that lives within. The warfare continues until some part of us steps up and is willing to forgive. Our well-being depends on it.

Forget past mistakes. Forget failures. Forget everything except what you're going to do now and do it.

WILLIAM C. DURANT

BRIDGETT'S STORY

Let me listen to me and not them.

GERTRUDE STEIN

It is typical to feel tired and stressed when you're twenty-two years old and going through finals week at the close of your second year of college. That's why Bridgett avoided going to the doctor for as long as she could. Plus, she didn't like going to doctors. Eventually, however, her fatigue was too much, and in April 2007, she finally went for a checkup.

The news was harsh. She had stage 3 non-Hodgkin's lymphoma. There was no sugarcoating from the doctor who delivered the news. "This is very aggressive," he prophesized, "and you'll probably die in six months."

No wonder she didn't like doctors.

Bridgett was so terrified that she chose not to share the news with anyone except her best friend, Apryl, with whom she lived. Urgently, and together, they researched the disease and at last got a second opinion.

Test results showed that Bridgett's disease was progressing. The cancer had wrapped around her ovaries and ran up her back. It was also evident in her throat.

Treatment options were laid out: chemo and radiation.

"I'm not a fan of chemo and radiation," Bridgett shared with me. "I had seen what it has done to family members, and I didn't want to do it. But the doctors all agreed it was my best chance, so I began treatments in July. Just one round messed me up really badly. I'm petite and normally weigh 90 pounds, but with the chemo I couldn't eat anything, so I went down to 46 pounds."

She paused. "When I was supposed to start my second round, my doctor said she couldn't do it. She admitted that the chemo would kill me before the cancer would."

Meanwhile, Apryl hadn't given up her research and was looking for alternatives. She learned that Brenda Cobb, founder of the Living Foods Institute (LFI), was giving a lecture nearby. She coerced Bridgett into going.

Upon hearing Brenda's story about healing her own cancer by eating raw foods, Apryl thought this might be a second chance for Bridgett.

"I was willing to try anything, but I didn't have the money," Bridgett recalled. "Brenda offered us a two-for-one package, and even though Apryl and I still didn't have the money, we signed up for the class."

By then, the cancer had progressed to stage 4, and hospice had already been called twice. Bridgett's doctor told her nothing would help and that she had three weeks to live.

This was a turning point for Bridgett and the moment she took charge of her life. "When I heard that, I thought, 'No one can tell me how long I have to live!' I decided then and there I was going to the Living Foods Institute." She figured she had nothing to lose, and clearly her doctor had no better offers.

Bridgett, Apryl, and a few of their friends put on a fundraiser and finally raised enough money for the two friends to attend a January class at LFI. Apryl put Bridgett into the car and drove her from where they lived in Tennessee to Atlanta.

Bridgett felt peace the moment she walked into the Institute. "I knew that was exactly where I needed to be. Even if it was the end, it would be peaceful."

Bridgett and Apryl had enrolled in a ten-day program, but Bridgett spent the first three days sleeping on a couch at the back of the room. "People brought me food, and I'd throw it up. I coughed up blood; I was really weak. I did manage to do reflexology, and Brenda kept bringing me soup. When I was cold, they'd bring me blankets. Everyone was so nice."

Each day Bridgett felt a little better, and when the facilitator of the group started addressing emotional issues, Bridgett perked up. "I have a lot of mommy/daddy issues, and I began to work on them. Everyone there had some form of cancer, and we all went through the emotional work differently. Yet in a certain way, it was the same for all of us. I wanted mostly to let go of things. Issues from my past kept surfacing, and I kept letting them go. As I continued to detox, more issues would come up. I think putting good food in my body also helped me address the emotional stuff. I did a lot of forgiving—a lot.

"Pretty soon, I began to feel better. I was awake a little longer. One day, I broke out in hives because I was detoxing the chemo. Brenda and the other staff members were very reassuring and told me everything was OK."

Bridgett participated more and more deeply in the emotionally based processes. She developed severe headaches and didn't feel well. Even so, she recognized that she felt sick in a different way than she had before. "The days were long. We'd arrive at seven in the morning and stay until six in the evening. Yet I was really glad to be there. It was so positive. I was resting better and sleeping well.

"Then on day five, I was feeling strange, and I realized it was because I felt good! It was the first day in the past year I had woken up and didn't have to force myself out of bed. I took a shower without being wiped out. I spent the whole morning in the kitchen preparing food with everyone else. I drank some juices and didn't throw up. I took a shot of wheat grass and did an enema. I felt great through all of it!"

When she'd arrived at the LFI, Bridgett had been jaundiced. By the fifth day, normal color was returning to her face. On day seven, she walked several blocks to a nearby park and strolled around it. Every day she felt better, and every day she worked with the facilitator on the emotional issues left over from an abusive childhood. She continued to dig deep and forgive.

"By day ten, you would have thought I was twelve years old! I was jumping around, hopping and dancing. I knew my body was better. I knew it," she said.

Bridgett didn't want to go home. She had found a safe haven and relished dwelling in the healing energy that elevated her. She did go home, but she reentered her life without many of the burdens she'd had in the past.

Three days after leaving the LFI, Bridgett visited the doctor who had told her she would be dead by that time.

"Everyone's jaws dropped when I walked in. I had gained 10 pounds. I was walking unattended. I was energized. They did a full blood panel—three times. After the third time, I asked what was going on. The blood panels had shown no evidence of cancer. My doctor was looking at a picture of the tumors in my lymph system, and then she looked at me and said, 'This is crazy. I'm your doctor, and I know you have cancer.'

"And I said, 'No, I don't.'

"This was so exhilarating! The cancer that had been tormenting my body was totally gone. I was finally normal.

"This doctor was really cool compared to other doctors I had seen. She wanted to know what I had done, but said it had to be off the record. She was blown away when I told her. She said it was frustrating not to be able to recommend LFI to others, because technically it's considered unethical to do that."

After receiving her clean bill of health, Bridgett went home and called both Brenda and the LFI facilitator who had worked with her on the emotional issues. The three of them cried tears of joy.

After hearing about her truly remarkable experience, I asked Bridgett what she thought had caused her cancer. She told me, "Before I went to Living Foods, I would've told you it was because of genetics and bad luck. But the truth is that I grew up in a negative and abusive home, and I did nothing but eat junk food—Cocoa Puffs and McDonald's—from the time I was a little kid until the day I went to the Institute. When I got to the Institute, I realized that I didn't think I was worthy of putting good food into my body. I learned about how I was thinking about myself, and I discovered all kinds of emotional garbage."

Vitamin D and Cancer

William B. Grant, PhD, has worked as a senior-level research scientist in the fields of laser remote sensing of the atmosphere and atmospheric sciences at SRI International, the Jet Propulsion Laboratory, and the NASA Langley Research Center. His career included pioneering laser-remote-sensing instrument development and participating on many NASA-led, airborne atmospheric-chemistry field missions. Dr. Grant is both the author and coauthor of more than two hundred papers and book chapters, 140 of which are related to health. He was elected fellow of the Optical Society of America in 1992.

Dr. Grant is currently the director of the Sunlight, Nutrition, and Health Research Center (sunarc.org), an entity devoted to research, education, and advocacy relating to the prevention of chronic disease through changes in diet and lifestyle. A foremost authority on the impact of vitamin D, he was kind enough to contribute the following information to this book.

***

Nearly thirty years ago, brothers Cedric and Frank Garland of Johns Hopkins University proposed the ultraviolet-B (UVB)/vitamin D/cancer hypothesis. A map of colon cancer mortality rates in the United States showed that the rate of colon cancer in the Northeast was approximately double that of the Southwest. As it is sunnier in the Southwest, they hypothesized that since the most important physiological effect of solar irradiance is production of vitamin D, it was likely that vitamin D reduced the risk of cancer.

For the two ensuing decades, science made slow but steady progress through a variety of ecological, observational, clinical, and laboratory studies pertaining to the relationship between vitamin D and cancer.

In 2000, when I was working as an atmospheric scientist for NASA, I came upon the updated *Atlas of Cancer Mortality Rates in the United States, 1950–94,* from the National Cancer Institute. Curious that many cancers, such as breast, colon, ovarian, and rectal cancer, had geographical patterns,[1] which by then had been found to be UVB sensitive, I obtained NASA satellite data on solar UVB doses at the earth's surface. I examined the correlation between solar UVB and cancer mortality rates, and identified about fourteen cancers that had mortality rates inversely correlated with solar UVB.

In 2002, my findings were published in the journal *Cancer*.[2] To extend the work, I added the influence of alcohol consumption and tobacco use, and examined the impact of Hispanic heritage, socioeconomic status, and urban/rural residence. After numerous rejections by medical journals, the new work was finally published in the periodical *Anticancer Research* in 2006.[3]

Observational studies support the use of vitamin D with breast and colorectal cancer, as well as non-Hodgkin's lymphoma and other cancers. There was a randomized controlled trial of 1,100 IU/day of vitamin D and 1,500 mg/day of calcium supplementation for postmenopausal women, which reported a 35 percent reduction in all cancer incidences from vitamin D and about 40 percent reduction from the calcium. It appears that it takes 1,000 to 4,000 IU/day of vitamin D to give up to a 50 percent risk reduction for many types of cancer and about a 25 percent reduction in all incidences of cancer. There have been numerous ecological, observational, and other studies of the theory.

Despite the growing evidence that vitamin D reduces the risk of cancer, the solar UVB/vitamin D/cancer hypothesis does not yet enjoy widespread acceptance. However, given the findings of additional beneficial effects for vitamin D in reducing the risk of several bacterial and viral infections, autoimmune diseases, cardiovascular diseases, and neurological diseases, including dementia, there is now greater interest in vitamin D from the public, health professionals, and health-policy leaders. To learn more, please visit s unarc.org.

Bridgett is the first to admit that dealing with the emotions behind her cancer was not easy. "At first, looking honestly at the emotional trauma that I had pent up in my body was scarier than thinking I was going to die of cancer. It's a very tough thing to let that stuff go. You have to take it one day at a time. You have to trust that you can let it go. Be delicate with yourself. It seemed like I'd take five steps forward and then three steps back. But I kept going. Now I say affirmations every day. Anytime I have a flood of emotion that upsets me, I'll take a moment, excuse myself from the situation, and go journal, journal, journal."

Bridgett's zest for life was vibrating through the phone line. "I'm a strong woman now. I'm not who I used to be. I look at what upsets me, and I move through it so that I can keep moving forward." Bridgett also practices yoga and maintains a diet that is 80 percent raw.

Perhaps the most surprising part of her story is the relationship she now has with her parents. "Even though they supported me as much as they could when I was sick, we never had a good dynamic. If anything, the whole cancer episode opened a door for us to have a new type of relationship. Now they're more like friends than parents. One of the things I came to understand was that I would never have a good parent-child relationship with them. I accept them the way they are. I'm loving getting to know them as an adult."

Other dynamics have changed in her life as well. "When I got back from Atlanta, some of the people who gave money for the fundraiser didn't believe that I had really been as sick as I was because they couldn't believe the turnaround in my health. They thought I had scammed the whole thing for the money. I guess some people don't want to accept that they can do something that positive for themselves and make such a big change."

When we spoke, Bridgett was planning a move to Los Angeles, where Apryl lives. She plans to pursue a career in acting, and she sees this move as another one of the positive changes that came from her near-death experience. "I live from strength now.

I'm so much more independent. I value life. Before, I took so much for granted. There are things I want to do in life, and I'm no longer waiting for them to happen to me. I have to go for it.

"I also appreciate people more. And I love myself. It's good to love yourself and take care of yourself first."

Bridgett's experience has done more than relieve her of cancer. She had also had a lifetime of poor vision and allergies, and now she no longer wears corrective lenses and no longer suffers from allergies.

She no longer sees a doctor. "I totally believe that we all have the ability to heal ourselves. I wake up every morning and say, 'Thank you! I have another day of being healthy!'"

Forgiveness is the economy of the heart ... forgiveness saves the expense of anger, the cost of hatred, the waste of spirits.
HANNAH MORE

BRENDA COBB

The Living Foods Institute

Author of *The Living Foods Lifestyle*

None of us will ever accomplish anything excellent or commanding except when he listens to this whisper which is heard by him alone.
RALPH WALDO EMERSON

Brenda Cobb's life story is a tour de force. If Hollywood picked it up, surely the finest actresses would vie for the part. That's because Brenda's story presents a whole new version of the familiar "riches to rags to riches" plotline. Additionally, as is true for everyone with the wisdom to make it so, getting cancer was the catalyst that spurred her to live her life fully and devote herself to helping others do the same.

Let's start with when she was diagnosed with breast and cervical cancer in 1999. "I was flabbergasted," she said. "Compared to other people, I ate well. I also had a successful business, and this wasn't in my plans."

Her plans were embedded in being the successful owner of an Atlanta-based film and television production company and talent agency. She produced big shows, at times shooting events of more than fifty thousand people that were later translated into nearly thirty different languages. She was the quintessential Type A personality.

"By that time, I had become very powerful. I was a leader in the industry, and I had won a lot of contracts. But I was also hardened and ruthless to the people who worked for me. If someone didn't do something right, I'd scream and yell, and then I'd fire them. I figured I was in it to be successful, so if they weren't there to do exactly what I wanted, they were history."

Her hard shell was badly shaken after the diagnosis. She had watched her mother, her aunts, and other family and friends with female cancers suffer the traumas of mastectomies, hysterectomies, chemotherapy, and radiation. Then she watched them die, either from the treatments or from a cancer that returned with a vengeance.

"I didn't want to go through that," Brenda recalled with a fast-paced Southern accent. "I was sobbing. I told my doctor, 'I'm not going to do what you want me to.'

"He asked me, 'Then what are you going to do?' I told him I didn't know. He said that if I didn't do what he suggested, I'd be dead in six months."

Instead, she prayed. "I knew what I *wasn't* going to do. I saw what those treatments did to others and then how they didn't work, so I prayed for God to please show me what I *could* do. And a little voice inside said, 'Go to the health food store.'"

When she arrived at the store, the clerk showed her a book called *How I Conquered Cancer Naturally* by Eydie Mae. "I touched it and got cold chills all over my body. The book was speaking to me. That was it. I read it, and it completely made sense to me. It was like coming home again."

That's when Brenda's new job began, which was to do everything she could to heal her cancer with natural methods. She began by learning about the work of Ann Wigmore, considered the "mother of living foods" and an expert on using raw and living foods to cleanse and heal. Then she learned about the cleansing benefits of enemas and wheatgrass implants.

"The more I cleansed my body, the more I found myself dealing with repressed emotional issues. In fact, as time went on, the emotional component of my journey really became the focal point of my overall healing. Eating living foods, working with essential oils and herbs, doing the wheatgrass implants—all that was important. But the emotional healing, that's what was truly at play."

As Brenda unearthed her buried emotional life, she began to piece together how she had gotten cancer. "It was all about anger. I was angry at my mother from my childhood. I remembered that she had given my dog away, and I liked my dog more than I liked my mother. But I was mostly angry with the men in my life, starting with my father. He was a wonderful father; I loved him, but he had negative issues about his own self-worth. He was an alcoholic, very dysfunctional. I became aware of all kinds of rage I had toward him. I was angry with my ex-husband and many times even wished he were dead."

Before she started the production company, Brenda also had a business partner with whom she shared a successful interior design firm. She trusted her partner and had given herself completely to the success of the business. But he hadn't been the man he made himself out to be, and the company went bankrupt.

"I lost my home and my car. I became enraged. I hated him. This was after my first husband and I had split, which also brought up anger in me because I kept thinking, 'Another man screwed me over! Another one!'"

After that experience, Brenda told herself that she was on her own, that she had to become totally independent, and that she could rely on no one. The idea was easy to grasp—even familiar. Ever since she was young, Brenda had been an A-student, an overachiever, a self-motivated go-getter who had gotten what she wanted. As a young woman, she competed in beauty pageants.

"There was something within me that *had* to win—and I did. There were other girls who were much prettier, much more talented than I, but I *knew* the crown was mine. I just *knew.* I'd go to bed the night before a pageant and practice my winning speech. There was no other option. When I decided to go it alone in business, it was like the anger was saying, 'I'll show you. I can do it better without you!' It fueled me so that I couldn't fail."

She tapped that same dogged determination in order to heal. "I believed in it. I had faith. I never doubted it—*ever.* I knew enough to know that I was going to heal. If there were people around who didn't want to support me, I'd tell them to leave me alone. That's why I healed so quickly and so well. I completely surrendered to it. If you can get to that point, instantaneous healing can occur because you fully accept and believe in your healing. When you doubt it, it sets up an acidic reaction in your body. It cancels out what works. I tapped into the same thing that made me know I'd win the crowns in those beauty pageants."

Healing didn't come without vigorous and devoted work of forgiving the people in her life whom she felt had wronged her, including herself. She found deep liberation after reading Colin Tipping's *Radical Forgiveness,* and Louise Hay's *You Can Heal Your Life.* She also took responsibility for whatever she was experiencing in life.

"As I went through my emotional healing, the hardness in me dissolved. I became sweeter, kinder, softer, gentler, more loving, more compassionate, and more helpful. I no longer raised my voice when I didn't get what I wanted. I recognized that I truly am a spiritual being inhabiting a human body. Every lesson I've gone through has helped me learn more."

Six months after her diagnosis, and in the very time frame that her doctor had told her she'd be dead, Brenda went back to her doctor for a checkup. She was cancer free.

With the confirmation of radiant health, Brenda experienced an overwhelming desire to open a center where she could help people by teaching them about the healing approach that had worked so well and so quickly for her. "My whole life was taken over by a higher mission. With the help of my son and my husband, I began the living foods lifestyle in February 1999 and by June, I was offering my first class on raw and living foods."

Since then, thousands of people have attended her ten- or twelve-day intensive course at the Living Foods Institute, while hundreds of thousands have listened to her lecture or have attended shorter workshops and seminars. She's also written or coauthored more than ten books, including *The Living Foods Lifestyle,* for which the doctor who issued her death sentence wrote the foreword. He is now practicing the raw foods lifestyle.

According to Brenda, "Everyone would love an instant fix, the magic bullet. I wish I could say that drinking wheatgrass would heal everything. But it's really all about energy. You set up an energetic pattern by the way you think, what you put into your body, and what you take out of your body."

She provided an example of how true that statement is. For several years, she experienced shoulder pain so severe that she couldn't raise her hand above her head. She saw acupuncturists and chiropractors, but nothing worked. Someone suggested that she have an *energy treatment,* where the energetic blocks causing the problem are removed.

"I didn't know anything about energy treatments, but I was desperate. What the practitioner told me was that my shoulder pain wasn't from an injury. Rather it was from stuff about my mother being controlling, narrow-minded, and manipulative. I was carrying the energetic in my shoulder. As the practitioner cleared the block, she told me how I could change my thinking, forgive my mother, and let it go. She told me that I didn't have to please my mother anymore, that I could do things without her approval, and that although I couldn't change her, I could change my thoughts around her. Two days later, I was able to raise my arm over my head.

"That was an aha moment. I didn't understand what she'd done, but it worked. So I started bringing people like that into the Institute. Now we're seeing serious metastasized cancers and other diseases healing very quickly. But it's not just by eating raw foods for two weeks. The people who experience 'miracles' are the ones who change their energetic field."

Not only are people just energy, according to Brenda, but food also carries a vibration, an energy, that has a domino effect. "When you're eating living, sprouted foods and getting the benefit of their enzymes and nutrients, you're directly connecting to the spiritual vibration of the food, and your thoughts are raised. When your mental and emotional fields are elevated, your physical body will also heal."

She summed it up like this: "We make healing about empowerment. We do that in a hands-on, fun, and exciting atmosphere. Students learn not to dread what they can't do. Instead, they learn to focus on what they can do to take care of themselves. Not only do they learn how to prepare the very best food for their bodies, but they also begin to access a deeper understanding of who they are and what they're capable of.

You can learn a lot in a ten- or twelve-day course, but that's just the beginning."

The Particulars

Where: Atlanta, Georgia

Who: Brenda Cobb no longer facilitates the courses because her career has taken her on the road and before the computer to write more books. A number of competent, passionate, loving, and devoted staff members teach the material, offer hands-on recipe-preparation classes, and provide healing "treatments." The kitchen is also staffed by a loving passel of volunteers who do the lion's share of chopping, juicing, soaking, and preparing the foods that go into the class-made recipes.

What to expect: Classes start at 8:00a.m., at which time everyone is served freshly pressed wheatgrass juice. Participants then congregate in the industrial-sized kitchen, don their hairnets, and learn exactly how to prepare different raw foods recipes. At the same time, people come and go from the kitchen so they can engage in a "treatment," such as reflexology, colonics, Indian head massage, spiritual readings, Bach Flower Remedy treatments, and more. By noon, class members are eating the food they have prepared.

Afternoons consist of group activities, such as lectures from the facilitator, informative movies, or demonstrations from visiting practitioners. There is general sharing by volunteers and daily affirmations. Class is dismissed around 6:00 p.m.

Where to stay: The Institute provides a list of local hotels, bed-and-breakfasts, or other lodging options and will help book all your travel arrangements.

Cost: $1,800 to $4,900 for the ten- and twelve-day programs, and for those who would like to teach others, $12,900 for the Educator Certification Course.

Who goes: People come from all over the world. Many have cancer, diabetes, heart disease, obesity, multiple sclerosis, Parkinson's, lupus, and more. Some who come are healthy and want to stay in good health and prevent future problems. Others want to reverse and slow the aging process or become raw and living foods chefs.

Contact Information:

livingfoodsinstitute.com
404-524-4488
800-844-9876

Love is an act of endless forgiveness, a tender look which becomes a habit.

PETER USTINOV

CHAPTER 3

Meaning

Truth, like gold, is to be obtained not by its growth, but by washing away from it all that is not gold.
LEO TOLSTOY

I believe that acquiring cancer, or any other disease, has meaning. Even though our first response is often to shout that we are victims of a random universe (because we certainly don't deserve this stuff!), to me, there is a design behind all of it that can be very difficult, but not impossible, to discern. Unless we're blessed with a blast of Divine insight, discovering the meaning—which is usually a totally subjective experience—calls for intense and honest internal inquiry.

At first, I found only unanswerable questions. My friend Janine, a hard-core bicyclist and equestrian, died of lung cancer in her late thirties. She had never smoked. Meanwhile, other people suck down two packs a day and live until they are ninety. Why do animals get cancer? Why, most especially, do children get cancer? What could possibly be the meaning of that? Is the food we eat and the air we breathe so filled with toxins now that none of us are immune?

So far, science has been unable to solve the mystery of cancer. Sure they know that smoking, poor eating habits, and at times genetics are related to certain cancers, but why doesn't everyone who smokes or regularly chows down on saturated fat end up with the disease? Why does one person with a history of cancer in the family get it, while others in the family do not?

Even though my first diagnosis left me reeling, the second one brought home the belief that all things happen on purpose and that we do not live in a random universe. I could no longer ignore the fact that this disease was somehow mine, and that it was happening (again) for a reason. I wasn't comfortable living out my experience without at least some glimmer of understanding the purpose behind it.

Seeking answers motivated me to turn to my internal environment. The veils of uncertainty began to lift as I accepted that fear and mistrust were ubiquitous characters ingrained in the fabric of my daily thoughts. I saw how I had grown so accustomed to my subtle strain of fear that I accepted it as a normal part of the architecture of my everyday life. But the influence of fear and mistrust was so deeply hidden and insidious that not even my closest friends knew that they shadowed me. The truth was only mine to deny and camouflage, and eventually, to embrace and release.

I began to cleanse myself of grievances from throughout my life, and soon clearly perceived a link between the pollution of my perceived world and the deteriorating cells in my body.

As time went on, I laid the paving stones for how I could live with and give meaning to adversity. They included:

- **Accepting the situation.** Giving up resistance to what is; giving up whatever I was fighting against and giving my energy instead to clarifying what I wanted. On some days, that meant being present or patient; on other days, it meant finding the right way to relieve pain. Overall, it meant becoming well.

- **Surrendering.** This wasn't about giving up or failing. Surrendering meant allowing the Divine intelligence within to take over and guide me. Surrendering opened my heart to new ways of being and to continually accepting that what showed up could impart meaning that I may have missed before. Surrender meant allowing what came forth, and proceeding in peace and hope rather than in anger, apathy, or resignation.
- **Forgiving.** This added up to forgiving myself, others, God, even life itself. I had to forgive everything. Forgiveness became central to my healing, and to my being able to recognize and trust the bigger story that was playing out.
- **Being grateful.** Once I quit seeing what I lacked and instead realized

the abundance of blessings that surrounded me, it was no longer difficult to find meaning. I looked around and was in awe at the beauty all around me. Every day, I take note of what I have. I do my best to dwell in joyous appreciation.

- **Delivering myself to love.** This has a double meaning. It was, and continues to be, a request to both give and receive love. Being within both the giving and receiving ends of love is healing. Love is at the heart of what it's all about.

My life improved dramatically after I created this paradigm, but then I was sideswiped with the third diagnosis.

The prognosis was terrifying. I lost sight of all hope—until I decided that I possessed something within that was bigger than the cancer. I decided I had what it took to keep going. I decided I had to save myself. How I would do it remained uncertain, but by giving myself entirely to the loving wonders and mystery of this universe we occupy, I knew that I would.

I dove in head first. My diet changed, my focus became clearer than ever before. I would find the power to heal, but to do that, I knew I had to commit myself to an even deeper ferocity and dedication. I knew that I must descend into the dark, intimidating basement of my mind. It was time to shed light on the subconscious thoughts and beliefs that might be feeding my fears and creating self-sabotaging outcomes—elements that could be impacting my cells.

Shame is perhaps the most destructive of emotions and I knew I had to free myself of it. Without shame, it's not so difficult to look at your dark side. In my case, I was much more afraid of dying and leaving behind my two children than being ashamed of what I might learn about myself. I wanted to know everything. I still do.

During many remarkable months of eating only living foods and cleansing myself of lifeless thoughts and emotions, I felt better than I ever had before or since. A real and certain transformation occurred. I metamorphosed into the magnificence of who I am, and who all of us really are. All because of cancer.

I got it.

I got cancer so I could become whole. I knew that even with another diagnosis, nothing could rob me of the beauty of that experience, nor the freedom of living without fear and mistrust, nor the peace of knowing the healing and transcendent power of love.

Someday, I will die. But I will have lived my life with the understanding of what it means to be physically, mentally, and spiritually whole. I will die having solved the most challenging personal mystery of my life, which isn't "Why did I get cancer?" but rather "Who am I and why am I here?"

The meaning of your cancer can only be explored subjectively. You will likely be discouraged from seeking meaning by your caring doctors and loving friends or family. Most will promise that there is no discernable reason why you got the disease. Most will want to protect you from going on a wild-goose chase. Their intentions are good. Still, if in your heart you want to excavate what the disease may mean in relation to you, then only you can decide if seeking answers is a worthy pursuit.

If you bring forth what is within you, what you bring forth will save you. If you do not bring forth what is within you, what you do not bring forth will destroy you.
THE GOSPEL OF THOMAS

GINNY'S STORY

Within us all there are wells of thought and dynamos of energy which are not suspected until emergencies arise.
THOMAS J. WATSON

Ginny's first experience with cancer was in 1994. She visited four different doctors before finding out that the mole on her arm was indeed a melanoma.

After a wide incision removed a large chunk from her arm, Ginny reassured herself that everything would be fine. She took extra vitamin C and went on with her busy life in London as a consultant and a coach.

Three years later, she discovered a lump under her arm. It turned out that cancer had developed in her lymph nodes close to where the original melanoma had been. It wasn't widespread, but Ginny decided this time that she would do something more proactive. She decided to follow the Gerson Therapy (a nutritional program) for eighteen months. She wasn't having CT scans at the time, but everything was fine for the next five years. (Note: For more information on the Gerson Therapy, see section "CHARLOTTE GERSON".)

In 2001, she began having trouble with her vision. Her eyelids became droopy, and she was extremely fatigued. She tried to ignore the visual disturbances, but they were distressing. So she finally went to a doctor. He diagnosed her with myasthenia gravis, a chronic, progressive autoimmune disorder characterized by chronic fatigue and muscular weakness, especially in the face and neck.

Shortly after, Ginny went to Findhorn, a spiritual community in northern Scotland. She was excited to be there, but had no energy to do the work she intended to do. She was feeling antisocial and only wanted to sleep. At that point, she decided to investigate what was going on within her body. When she returned to London, she requested a brain scan. The film showed a tumor in her brain, and further scans showed multiple tumors in her lungs, spleen, and stomach.

"I was totally freaked out," Ginny reported. "I asked the doctor how long I had to live and was told six months.

"I was in shock. They put me on high doses of steroids. I decided to go to the annual spiritual retreat I often went to in California. I shared my situation with my teacher, John-Roger. He spoke to me, shared some wisdom, and held my head in his hands. I started swelling up, and my face looked like a chipmunk's. It was very difficult. But I was given so much love and support there, it gave me the strength to go on."

When she got home, Ginny began investigating possible treatments. She knew she would undergo brain radiotherapy. In addition, she and her friends spent hours researching what else might help. Her only symptom was fatigue, but she powered through it as she scoured the Internet. Meanwhile, the steroids gave her a ravenous appetite and made her speedy, so she didn't sleep well. Soon other side effects from the steroids began to kick in.

"You swell up. It's hideous. Friends didn't even recognize me. I didn't look anything like me. I was bald, wearing an eye patch, and I had gotten fat from the drugs. My left eye was fine, but my right eye couldn't focus.

"My friends and I diligently sought alternative treatments, but there didn't seem to be anything that could help. Even the people at the Gerson Institute said they couldn't help." Other well-known alternative centers in the US also turned her away. She became desperate.

Meanwhile, Ginny underwent radiotherapy on her brain, which wiped her out for two solid weeks. She lost most of her hair, and an area of it has never fully grown back because the roots were destroyed. After absorbing all the radiation her brain could endure, Ginny began working with Dr. Etienne Callebout, a naturopathic oncologist based in the United Kingdom (see appendix for contact information). Dr. Callebout is a medical doctor, but he is also trained in naturopathic and homeopathic medicine, acupuncture, and nutritional therapies.

"Basically," Ginny said, "he travels around the world going to conferences and acquiring information from little-known doctors or healers who've had success. He's also part of MedInsight, a group that studies new pharmaceutical drugs that could work for cancer. He's incredibly clever and very wide-reaching in his research."

Dr. Callebout put Ginny on an intense regimen of five freshly pressed vegetable juices per day, three coffee enemas per day, and literally hundreds of supplements. He also instructed her to soak her feet in a bucket of very hot water that contained mustard and cayenne, while at the same time holding a hot water bottle to her liver and cold packs on the back of her neck.

"The purpose of all this was to stimulate my system, to increase my metabolic rate. I'd do a liver flush every four weeks, two-week juice fasts, three weeks on supplements. I was doing a major detox and giving massive support to my immune system."

A month after she completed radiation, Ginny visited her mainstream doctor again. A brain scan showed that nothing had changed; the brain tumor was still present, and the size had not changed. Ginny remembered, "It was a horrible moment. My friend and housemate, Stacey, who had been taking care of me, was with me, and we began to laugh hysterically. Nothing had changed. We had done so much, and it was so awful that all we could do was laugh."

Ginny couldn't tolerate any more radiation, so there was nothing the doctors could do. They requested that she return in two weeks for another scan.

Ginny maintained the protocol that Dr. Callebout had assigned her. Stacey continued to chop vegetables, press juice, prepare enemas, and count out her supplements. "Stacey doesn't like vegetables. She never eats them, but she prepared them for me every day. I couldn't have done it without her."

Two weeks later, and after the next scan, the brain tumor had diminished in size. What surprised her oncologist, however, was that the tumors in her body were also much smaller—even though they had not been treated with radiation. The doctor was amazed at the development and asked Ginny what she had been doing. Upon hearing Ginny's description, the doctor lost interest.

German New Medicine

Tracing Emotional Trauma as the Starting Point of Cancer

German-born Dr. Ryke Geerd Hamer spent years in charge of cancer patients at the University Clinic in Tübingen, while also running a private practice with his wife, Dr. Sigrid Hamer. Eventually they moved to Italy, where Dr. Hamer realized his goal of treating the sick in the slums of Rome free of charge. Shortly after their relocation, the Hamers' son, Dirk, was accidentally shot and critically injured. Three months later, nineteen-year-old Dirk succumbed to the injuries and died in his father's arms.

Shortly after Dirk's death, Dr. Hamer was diagnosed with testicular cancer. Since he had never been seriously ill, he postulated that the development of his cancer could be directly related to the unexpected loss of his son. Dirk's death, and his own experience with treating cancer, set Dr. Hamer on an extraordinary scientific journey.

After his son's death, he returned to Germany. As the head internist of a cancer clinic at the University of Munich, Dr. Hamer began to investigate his cancer patients' histories and soon learned that, like him, they all had experienced an unexpected shock of one sort or another. But he took his research even further. Pursuing the hypothesis that all bodily events are controlled from the brain, he analyzed his patients' brain scans and compared them with their corresponding medical and psychological records. To his amazement, he found a clear correlation between certain "conflict shocks," how these shocks manifested on the [cancerous] organ, and how all these processes are connected to the brain. Until then, no studies had examined the [possible] origin of the disease and the role of the brain as the mediator between the psyche and a diseased organ.

Dr. Hamer discovered that every disease originates from a shock or trauma that catches us completely by surprise. The moment the unexpected conflict occurs, the shock strikes a specific area in the brain (later called Hamer Focus, or HH, from the German phrase *Hamerscher Herd)* visible on a brain scan as a set of sharp concentric rings.

The brain cells that receive the conflict impact send a biochemical signal to the corresponding body cells, causing the growth of a tumor, a meltdown of tissue, or functional loss, depending on which brain layer (the endoderm, mesoderm, or ectoderm) receives the shock.

Over the years, Dr. Hamer has been able to confirm his discoveries with over forty thousand case studies.

The result of his scientific work is the "Psyche-Brain-Organ" chart, which outlines the disease, the content of the biological conflict that causes it, where the corresponding lesion can be seen on a brain scan, how the disease manifests itself (the type of tumor) in the conflict active phase, and what can be expected in the healing phase.

Dr. Hamer's explanation of disease as a meaningful interplay between the psyche, the brain, and the corresponding organ refutes the view that disease occurs by chance or as a result of a mistake of nature. Based on sound scientific criteria, German New Medicine (GNM) shatters the myths of malignant cancer cells or destructive microbes, and identifies "infectious diseases" and cancerous tumors as natural biological emergency measures that have been in effect for millions of years and are designed to save the organism—not, as we have been taught, to destroy it. Under this enlightened view, diseases such as cancer lose their frightening image and can be recognized as meaningful, special, biological survival programs with which every human being is born.

To learn more about GNM, go to learninggnm.com.

Ginny continued with Dr. Callebout's treatment for a year. Her entire life was devoted to healing. She couldn't work, so Stacey took care of her. Ginny said, "It was such an incredible act of friendship and love. People ask, 'Wasn't it hard?' But it wasn't. We just got in this zone. We just did it. It was a weird time because I had a strange sense of peace. Stacey would say that I had a beatific smile on my face. I felt like I was being carried through the whole process, so it really wasn't hard.

"But there were some disgusting things I had to do. Drink clay in water and glasses of olive oil! Even now when I think of it, I retch. Stacey helped a lot. She'd cover up what I had to drink because it looked so gross! It was a very special time for our friendship. We really were in the zone."

By autumn 2002, Ginny had a complete remission of the tumors in her brain, lung, and spleen. The worst part of the experience, Ginny recalls, were the side effects from the steroids and the radiotherapy. "It seems like those treatments were worse than the cancer," she says. But once she was off the steroids, her energy returned.

I asked Ginny if she believes she's now cancer free. "That's a really good question. I don't go around proclaiming that, because I know there is always a possibility that it could return. But it has been over seven years now, and as time passes, the chance of a recurrence gets smaller and smaller. Most of the time I don't even think about it, but I guess it really has been an amazing recovery."

When I asked her what role her mind had played in either causing or healing her condition, Ginny had a lot to say.

"I don't know what proportion it played in the healing because I did so many things to get better. I had an unconscious determination that was a very natural thing. It wasn't forced.

That's what I mean when I say I was carried. There was no effort.

"As for what created it, I do subscribe to the theory that you experience a shock or disaster before the first onset of cancer. That had been the case for me with a very painful relationship split.

"I have received a great sense of strength from surviving cancer. I feel there is nothing that can really trip me up now. I'm much stronger. It's also really opened my heart. It may have been through being around Stacey and feeling her incredible love, and maybe also just the sense I had of being carried through it with a kind of spiritual loving. It was a really rich, profound, amazing experience."

Even though she sees a connection between the emotional trauma of that time and getting cancer, Ginny speaks strongly about the idea of not blaming yourself for getting the disease. "I hate the whole thing of 'How did you create your cancer?' There's a tyranny around the whole idea of positive thinking that people tend to use against themselves. Instead of positive thinking being a lovely tool, it becomes a stick that people beat themselves up with.

"At the same time, you must take responsibility for your healing. You must check out what's best for you. You have to stand up inside yourself and accept that you are the authority who will manage your own recovery."

Before her cancer experience, part of Ginny's work as a coach was assisting others with taking responsibility for their emotional state. Now she also works with people dealing with cancer, helping them cope with the emotional roller coaster and deepen their spiritual experience. She said, "My spiritual path played a huge part in getting better. In addition to that, my mother wrote to scores of monasteries, churches, and prayer communities asking them to pray for me. I'm a strong believer in the power of prayer, and I know that it can work. My Christian upbringing didn't go away through all this. It has strengthened, and my gratitude has deepened for my spiritual connection, especially with Jesus. I don't go to church, but my relationship has deepened. The entire experience made me stronger both emotionally and spiritually."

One of the outcomes of her journey is that Ginny is not afraid of dying. "While I was still going through my healing process, I had a conversation with a friend. We were talking about what could happen. We talked about the fact that when you really face death, despite the fear that this acceptance might somehow hasten death, the opposite occurs. It was as though by accepting that I could die—and by doing all the completions that this involved—somehow it liberated more energy for healing."

You can read more about Ginny's story and other stories she's written in *Integrative Cancer and Oncology News (ICON)* out of Great Britain (canceracti ve.com).

Start by doing what's necessary; then do what's possible, and suddenly you are doing the impossible.
ST. FRANCIS OF ASSISI

TIMOTHY C. BIRDSALL, ND, FABNO

Cancer Treatment Centers of America

Once the "what" is decided, the "how" always follows. We must not make the "how" an excuse for not facing and accepting the "what."
PEARL S. BUCK

By now, most people who watch television have seen advertisements for Cancer Treatment Centers of America (CTCA). The ads do a good job. They feature sad and desperate people, who have been told there's nothing more to do for their cancer, transforming into smiling, hopeful people upon speaking with a doctor from one of the five CTCA campuses.

Because of CTCA's huge public relations budget and ads that pulled a little too hard on my heartstrings, I admit to having been suspicious of its real deal. Was it just another chain of hospitals with Big Pharma paying the bills, luring more desperate cancer patients through their doors? Or did they really offer something different?

After my conversation with Dr. Timothy Birdsall, a naturopathic doctor (ND) and vice president of Integrative Medicine for the CTCA enterprise, I was grateful that I could welcome it in this book. The centers do indeed function as hospitals, but they offer much more than abbreviated visits with oncologists and a narrow menu of conventional treatment options.

According to Dr. Birdsall, what sets CTCA centers apart from other cancer treatment centers is that they put patient needs first, which inevitably includes providing emotional and spiritual counseling and incorporating alternative care into therapeutic programs.

"We are only and always about what's best for the patient," Dr. Birdsall told me from his office in Phoenix. "Everyone in health care says that, but the sad reality is that few places actually do it. Most of the large facilities that deal with cancer are academic medical centers. They focus on educating students, and they engage in medical research. But patient care often comes last. Even in the community setting, virtually all hospitals are referral driven. So, for example, the doctor admits the patient into the hospital, so the doctor is really the hospital's client, not the patient. Then the insurance companies pay the bills, so they're also the client rather than the patient. In fact, the patient frequently isn't even in the dialogue."

So how did a healthcare organization that really and truly wanted to work with patients as its primary concern come into being? Someone with a personal experience of cancer decided to change things: Richard J. Stephenson, owner of CTCA.

Mr. Stephenson owned a different hospital before founding CTCA, so as a businessman, he was already aware of and working in the health care industry. He was also interested in alternative health care. When his mother got cancer, he was appalled by how she was treated at a local cancer facility and the lack of options available to her. After she died, he vowed he would do something about it.

The first CTCA hospital opened in 1988 in Zion, Illinois. Treatments there include a robust list of integrative choices: intensive nutritional intervention, naturopathic treatments, mind-body medicine and healing techniques, acupuncture, chiropractic, and more. An aggressive oncology-rehabilitation department offers physical therapies, occupational therapies, and exercise facilities. Pastoral care and spiritual support are also offered.

The success of Stephenson's flagship hospital enabled him to open other centers. Now CTCA centers can also be found in Tulsa, Philadelphia, Seattle, and Phoenix. The Stephenson family still owns the hospitals as a for-profit corporation. The fact that CTCA is thriving says more to Dr. Birdsall about what it has to offer than anything else.

"Cancer is a complex disease that requires a wide array of medical and technological interventions to treat it successfully," Dr. Birdsall advised. "Naturopathic physicians alone can't do that. The patients need to be seen by all kinds of doctors—not only surgeons,

GI doctors, medical oncologists, radiation oncologists, but also naturopathic physicians, acupuncturists, chiropractors, and so on. Our hospitals are the only place in the country where all of those practitioners work under one roof."

Although the term "integrative medicine" has only been around since the early to mid-1990s, according to Dr. Birdsall, about three-quarters of cancer patients who come to CTCA are already using complementary medicine in an attempt to heal.

"We'd like to believe that all natural products are safe, but that's not true," he said. "Some products are fine to use together, but not all combinations of natural products and pharmaceutical drugs are appropriate. Invariably, when patients self-medicate, they increase the likelihood of a contraindication or interaction.

"We provide a care team that works together, knows each other, has common goals, and who are, therefore, able to make appropriate recommendations for everything from the best type of chemotherapy to homeopathic, herbal, and chiropractic treatment. It's unusual to have this kind of medical diversity among those who ordinarily don't even talk to each other. We meet three times a week to talk about what each patient needs and to construct their treatment plan in a truly interdisciplinary fashion. In essence, we offer coordinated and appropriate care that doesn't exist anywhere else."

"What's more," said Dr. Birdsall, "each patient is evaluated for their unique nutritional needs once they understand and value the role that food plays in healing. Hospitals are famous for serving bad food. We do it differently. We have executive chefs at all our hospitals. We offer a range of food every day, including soup that's made fresh. We rarely cook things from a can or use something that's been frozen. It's more costly, but it's incredibly important. At the same time, we're aware that cancer treatments may affect appetites, so we're focused on palatability. We'll make special recipes if someone requests them."

With CTCA's holistic approach, I asked Dr. Birdsall if it offered anything for the emotional journey their patients are on. "The mind is enormously important with health and healing in general," he declared. "With cancer, one critical issue is helping patients find ways to process what's going on. They may be mourning the losses that have occurred since they've been ill. Just the word 'cancer' is frightening and oftentimes causes a huge amount of anxiety. We know that anxiety and depression impair immune function. The solution isn't to say, 'Don't be depressed.' That only adds to the problem. It's really a matter of figuring out appropriate strategies for leveraging the power of the mind in order to stimulate the immune system."

To that end, CTCA provides psychotherapists and various therapies to help with emotional issues. For some people, it might be talk therapy, while others might do well with relaxation or breathing techniques, biofeedback, or regaining a sense of power by defining life goals and plans.

Birdsall said these services don't come out of the blue. They're researched. "We want to know that we're delivering what patients tell us they value. We want to know that we're delivering our promise to our patients."

To ensure that it is, Dr. Birdsall explained that CTCA has adopted a system of evaluation similar to the one used in four- and five-star hotels. The point is to keep track of how satisfied their patients are with the service they received at the hospitals, and if the levels are low, to then correct the problem.

Not only is CTCA keeping track of patient satisfaction, but it's also keeping tabs on the quality of its patients' lives, in addition to their survival rates. Dr. Birdsall claimed that employing naturopathic doctors as part of the treatment team has been highly beneficial, especially when it comes to pain management and fatigue treatment. Pancreatic cancer patients, for example, report experiencing far less pain and fatigue than those without the remedies of the NDs. They also live longer than patients in other cancer centers or in clinical trials. There's similar data on colon and lung cancer patients. "The types of things we're doing compared to other approaches are overwhelmingly good," Birdsall claimed.

Even though each of the five CTCA hospitals boasts the same level of customer satisfaction, they do not offer the same treatments. For example, the center in Chicago has a specialty center that focuses on blood cancers and stem cells, while the Seattle center offers outpatient services only. This means that if you live in Phoenix and have a certain type of leukemia, you might be sent to Chicago, at least for your initial evaluation, even though there's a CTCA center in Phoenix.

In essence, while each hospital has specific areas of unique expertise, they all provide comprehensive cancer care for virtually all types of adult cancers. Since about 50 percent of the patients who come to CTCA have advanced and complex types of cancers, Dr. Birdsall believes it's the right way to do business.

"There are no hard-and-fast rules about why and when we advise that you go to another center; we just want you to get the best possible treatment. So if that means sending you out of state, we'll do it. We all work together and utilize the same electronic medical-record system, so going back and forth between hospitals won't be a problem."

Given his holistic approach to dealing with cancer, I wanted to know Dr. Birdsall's take on what causes cancer. I was delighted by his response, because I had heard these words only from the mouths of two other alternative doctors, never someone in a more conventional setting.

"There is no such thing as 'cancer.' I wish the word didn't even exist. It implies a single condition, and there are over two hundred different diseases that we call cancer. They may have some features in common, but they have many differences. And they are all caused by different things." He said, "Take lung cancer. Eighty percent of the time, it's caused by smoking. That means we could potentially eradicate 80 percent of the cases if no one ever smoked again. We wouldn't eliminate it completely, but there would be a dramatic difference. Simple. Not so with other cancers.

"Cancer is a result of a whole succession of genetic changes and damage. The damage can be caused by myriad influences. They're now saying it takes five, ten, or twenty genetic hits to create a cancer cell. Unfortunately, the chances of getting cancer increase as you get older. The good news is that we're living longer because we've learned to prevent other diseases from killing us sooner. The bad news is that we're living long enough to get cancer.

"We've got long-term exposure to low levels of toxins all the time—the pollution in our water, air, and food, as well as pesticides, lead, industrial solvents, and chemicals. That's one big long hit, which I think is as bad as twenty smaller hits. Even though DDT was banned nearly forty years ago, it's still detectible in the average adult. It's in our food chain.

"When a cell is pre-cancerous, your tumor-suppressor genes are supposed to kick in to either repair the damage or destroy the defective cell. But if the gene that's supposed to protect you is damaged, now you have two damaged cells that can't self-destruct. That ramps up the cellular production, and it gets out of control.

"So when people ask, 'Will we find a cure to cancer?' I say no, because there are too many different diseases, and there isn't a single answer that will ever cure them all."

Meanwhile, Dr. Birdsall and his colleagues continue to work on treating most cancers in an innovative and comprehensive manner.

The Particulars

Where: Zion, Illinois (96 beds); Tulsa, Oklahoma (48 beds); Philadelphia, Pennsylvania (42 beds); Seattle, Washington (outpatient only); and Phoenix, Arizona (24 beds).

Who: There are 100 to 150 physicians on staff and many more acting as consultants. This adds up to well over 400 doctors enterprise-wide.

What to expect: When you call, you'll talk to a real live person, 24/7, 365 days a year. (If you get voice mail, it's at a peak moment.) The Oncology Information Specialist will provide information about the kinds of treatment options that might be available and where to go, but cannot diagnose. Upon hanging up, callers should have a clear understanding of what their insurance will and will not cover. CTCA can help discern deductibles and co-pays. The Oncology Information Specialist will facilitate making appointments, which can usually be made immediately so callers can see a doctor within five to seven days.

Typical routine: Before the patient arrives, a nurse will call and review all their medical history. Medical records are sent prior to admission so that when the patient arrives, everything is ready. Once the patient arrives, the medical records are reviewed, typically with the same person the patient has already spoken to. Any additional tests or scans that might be needed will be scheduled right away. In addition to the oncologists, patients will see a naturopathic doctor, a dietician, and a mind-body therapist during their initial assessment. There's also a follow-up with an oncologist, where the treatment plan is presented and discussed in detail with the patient. If other medical issues come up, the center will invite in a specialist. Within three to four days of the patient seeing all the doctors and doing all the tests, a treatment plan is created with appropriate follow-up protocol.

Where to stay: All CTCA hospitals have some lodging onsite or close by, with additional arrangements with local hotels. The Arizona and Oklahoma centers have significant guest accommodations and shuttle service.

Cost: CTCA works with patients so they will know up front if Medicare will pay or how their insurance will contribute. Many services provided by CTCA, such as mind-body medicine, are not currently billed for because they are folded into overall treatment plans. CTCA does get some insurance reimbursement for nutritional and acupuncture treatments.

Miscellaneous: About 80 percent of the treatments at CTCA are done on an outpatient basis. Thousands of people visit the CTCA facilities each month. CTCA treats only adult patients with cancer; there are no pediatric facilities. All cancers are considered for treatment.

Contact Information:

Cancer Treatment Centers of America
14200 West Fillmore Street
Goodyear, AZ 85338
623-207-3371
cancercenter.com

*Once we believe in ourselves, we can
risk curiosity, wonder, spontaneous
delight, or any experience that reveals
the human spirit.*
E.E. CUMMINGS

JAMES GORDON, MD

Center for Mind-Body Medicine
Author of *Unstuck: Your Guide to the
Seven-Stage Journey Out of Depression*

***

*Pain is a part of being alive, and we
need to learn that. Pain does not last
forever, nor is it necessarily unbeatable,
and we need to be taught that.*

HAROLD KUSHNER

As a psychiatrist, James Gordon has a broad understanding of the value of treating cancer holistically. That includes providing emotional and spiritual support for sure, but he also embraces a strict regimen of exercise, detoxification, nutrition, and food as medicine, along with a range of complementary and alternative therapies.

This menu isn't your typical fare from a Harvard-trained doctor who also serves as a clinical professor in the departments of psychiatry and family medicine at Georgetown University School of Medicine. But this menu is in keeping with his posts as the dean of the Graduate College of Mind- Body Medicine at Saybrook University and as the chair of the White House Commission on Complementary and Alternative Medicine Policy.

Even with these credentials, it was more a personal interest in both cancer and cancer patients that inspired his current body of work. "I've been interested in working with cancer ever since I was a med student," he told me from his office in Washington, DC. "I was touched by the kids with cancer, but didn't do much with it because my work took me in other directions. Then I did some work with an adult who had brain cancer and had been through conventional treatment that didn't work. He asked me what thousands of people ask: 'What else can I do?'

In the 1970s, Dr. Gordon was using alternative treatments for himself, such as acupuncture, meditation, nutrition, and mind-body applications. The more he practiced what he learned from these modalities, the more he thought they might be able to offer something significant for people with cancer. When patients began asking what else they could do, he decided alternative treatments were worth pursuing.

"In the 1980s, it became clear that I was acting as a cancer guide to people who had been failed by conventional treatments, in addition to those who were using conventional treatments but were eager to learn about what else was available to help. Patients were responding well to the evidence-based guidance I was offering, and I realized there was a real need for this type of service."

By the early 1990s, Dr. Gordon was chairing the National Institutes of Health Office of Alternative Medicine—and 70 percent of the calls he received were inquiries about new ways of treating cancer. This, along with his personal experience as a cancer guide, stimulated Dr. Gordon to take the next step. He began to address the issue of creating new programs of integrative cancer care and providing information through the nonprofit Center for Mind-Body Medicine (CMBM), which he founded and currently directs. "My intention was to share with health care professionals and family caregivers, as well as cancer patients themselves, the best available information to help guide them through their cancer experience."

That vision led to the first Comprehensive Cancer Care (CCC) conference in 1998, to which almost one thousand patients, clinicians, researchers, policy makers, and patient-advocates came. In 2001, the Center for Mind-Body Medicine built on several years of CCC conferences and created CancerGuides, the world's only comprehensive training in integrative oncology.

"CancerGuides trains people how to integrate alternative treatments into the overall approach to healing. It equips both medical professionals and cancer patients to answer the question, 'What else can I do?' We teach our students to work with great sensitivity and to individualize the programs that can best help them through their experience. Over six thousand people came to our five Comprehensive Cancer Care conferences, and we've had over one thousand begin their training as cancer guides."

Deepak Chopra, Herbert Benson, Dean Ornish, Mehmet Oz, and Christiane Northrup endorse this work. Furthermore, CMBM offers professional training nationally in mind-body medicine and nutrition (food as medicine), as well as a program of global trauma relief based on the Center's practical model of self-awareness, self-care, and mutual help.

When asked about the role of the mind in contributing to and healing cancer, Dr. Gordon believes that not only is there a connection, but there is also evidence to support the effect of emotions and attitudes in people who've already been diagnosed with cancer.

"The connection between stress and the onset of cancer is weak scientifically," he said, "but it looks like it's there. We know that extreme stress over time significantly impairs immune function. Many people will tell you that they were under extreme stress before they got the disease—not all, but many.

"The effect of stress is significantly stronger once you've been diagnosed with cancer. We also know that those who deal with the disease optimistically do better, as do those who have a strong spiritual belief or who consider the cancer an opportunity for growth. People who become committed to their journey through and beyond cancer have a better quality of life and may live longer than those who don't possess those attributes."

Empirical evidence abounds that our minds and bodies are involved in a symbiotic dance and that mind-body approaches enhance immunity and improve quality of life. The studies on prolongation of life are far less consistent. Dr. Gordon referred to one study showing that women with breast cancer who participated in support groups lived longer than those who didn't. A subsequent study that replicated the first showed no increase.

"What's most outstanding from what I've seen is that people who see cancer as an opportunity for profound psychological and spiritual change seem to do better. There are lots of stories of people in denial who do well, but not as well as those who become engaged in their own healing process."

I asked Dr. Gordon if he believes the culture of cancer is changing. "More and more doctors in general, and oncologists in particular," he replied, "are realizing that there's a connection between the mind and body and that approaches other than the conventional may have something to offer. They come to the CancerGuides training we offer, and they see the possibilities! They read the studies and counsel their patients in a different, more open-minded way. I believe that in the future this comprehensive approach, which includes mind-body techniques and other evidence-based modalities, like nutrition, exercise, Chinese medicine, and support groups, will be part of everyone's care. We just need to give clinicians and patients an opportunity to look at the emerging facts through a new lens."

An ongoing obstacle to providing this type of care is that it's generally not reimbursable by insurance and doesn't fall within the training of oncologists. "Many oncologists have a hard time including non-pharmacological approaches or even looking at the evidence for alternative approaches. It's a challenge for them because they've been trained that it doesn't matter much. There's a disconnect. Even good nutrition isn't part of their belief system."

These hurdles don't stop Dr. Gordon from believing in the merit of integrating and *engaging* the mind to include alternative therapies in healing. "The change is slow, but it's real. When we began this work, there was only separation between conventional and alternative approaches. Now there is a Society for Integrative Oncology led by those who have worked with us on our programs, and the demand for CancerGuides is increasing each year."

Contact Information:

5225 Connecticut Ave. NW
Suite 414
Washington, DC 20015
202-966-7338

For more information on CancerGuides go to cmbm. org (click on "CMBM Certified Practitioners" to find a practitioner near you.)

For more information on or to contact Dr. Gordon, go to jamesgordon MD.com

He who cannot change the very fabric of his thought will never be able to change reality.

ANWAR AL-SADAT

CHAPTER 4

Authority

I was always looking outside myself for strength and confidence, but it comes from within. It is there all the time.
ANNA FREUD

A cancer diagnosis catapults us down a slippery, surreal chute into a world where we are stripped of power. The very word "cancer" frightens us, which explains why for years so many people refused to utter it.

These days a whole vocabulary propels the cancer culture and injects it with fear.

- **Prognosis:** Learned after sleepless nights of worst-case scenario fantasies while waiting for tests results.
- **Chemotherapy:** Poison that makes you bald, skinny, weak, and nauseated.
- **Radiation:** The same stuff that causes deformities after bombs are dropped, right? The same stuff from

the sun that *gives* you cancer, right?

- **Surgery:** Hospitals, needles, anesthesia, blood-pressure cuffs, catheters, beeping IV machines, drug-muffled pain.

Then we're bombarded with stories from well-meaning people who don't understand the trauma they're inflicting—stories about an uncle, a best friend's daughter, someone they knew and loved who died of cancer. Obliviously, they recount the horrific details of everyone they've ever known who has died of cancer—stories that deepen our feelings of powerlessness and cut a new notch of terror in our hearts.

Then there's the cancer environment—typically cold and clinical, with endless paperwork and where we tell our same story over and over and over again. Blood draws that leave tender bruises. The antiseptic smell. The cold, spotless linoleum floors upon which the shoes of medical personnel squeak—as though warning of danger—as they rush to their next powerless patient.

In truth, however, it's not the language or stories or environment of cancer that strips us of power. It's our *perception* that we have no power in cancer's world. It's especially pronounced if we are accustomed to a lifetime of giving our power to outside sources, which is the way many people live. It's a likely preference because it frees them from responsibility or blame.

Every day, in every single thing we do, we bow to authority of some kind or another. As children, we answered to our parents, teachers, and other adults. As we matured, we looked to peers for our sense of worth and belonging. When we began exploring our own authority, more often than not, we didn't trust it—and still don't. Why would we? Messages throughout our entire lives suggest that we don't possess the wisdom to know what's best. Rather than nurturing us to access, implement, and ultimately trust the innate wisdom within, our culture commands that we continue to look outside ourselves for what is real, true, and right.

This is especially true in the world of cancer. We've long been programmed to believe that doctors are the authority on health. True, they've studied disease for years and know far more than we do about the science and biology of what goes wrong. They're certainly versed on what drugs are most inclined to remedy the symptoms we present. Still, even with multiple medical degrees, they are *not* the authority on your cancer experience. You are.

To heal, you must embrace responsibility for yourself and take back your power. Be your own advocate, your own decision maker. Be the authority over your life experience and over every cell in your body.

When you are the authority, you go to a doctor to get a diagnosis. Then you have a series of discussions of possible treatments. Hopefully, he or she will be open to whatever options you are considering. It's good to get the doctor's point-of-view, because then you will know if it meshes with yours. Always remember: *you* decide whether the doctor before you is someone you can work with. *You* decide if he or she is recommending treatment options you believe in. If not, then go to another doctor. If that doctor doesn't do it, find yet another. *You* must be the authority that determines how you go about your cancer journey.

If you don't claim your authority during this most pivotal time of life, then you will be a perpetual victim (if the treatment fails) or randomly lucky (if it works). In either case, you remain a powerless pawn. In truth, you are *opting* for powerlessness by refusing to deliberately and consciously discern the best path for yourself.

I have several good friends who are doctors. They have educated me about the general mentality of the patients they see. "They want a quick fix," Paul tells me, his big brown eyes earnest and frustrated. "You tell them to change their eating habits or get more exercise, simple stuff that will take care of the problem, and they won't do it. They want a pill. Everybody wants a pill. Hardly anyone I treat is willing to take responsibility for their health."

When we relinquish responsibility (for anything), we believe it frees us from a burden. Someone else can handle it. Then if it goes wrong, we get to blame them. We don't have to take the rap. This very dynamic of foisting responsibility for life's challenges (including health) onto someone else is part of why we experience disease in the first place. Blame, resentment, fear, anger—these emotions are born of powerlessness. Only by embracing—taking responsibility for—the cancer and our healing do we fully reclaim our power and authority.

When we deeply consider the options before us, meditate on them, discuss them with our loved ones, and at last choose what's best, then we have the best chance to be at peace. That's the moment we become the authority on healing. Indeed, that's when we command it. And even if it doesn't work the way we want it to, we can't blame anyone, even ourselves, because there's no blame when we are true to the self. Indeed, blaming oneself is obsolete when choices come from true inner power and self-love.

During my first year of cancer, my radiologist and surgeon were at odds on how to perform follow-ups. The surgeon wanted to do a biopsy of the anal tissue, but my radiologist disagreed, saying that the biopsy incision would not heal since my skin had been so badly radiated. After listening to both sides, asking lots of questions, listening to my intuition, and talking it over with my husband, I decided to go with the radiologist.

The surgeon became agitated and rude, saying, "Well, let's just hope you don't come back to me next year with a new diagnosis that could have been prevented."

Jane, my family doctor, sided with the surgeon and took the insult even further: "So you live with a sore on your butt; it's better than the alternative. I mean, do you want to *stick around* or not?"

The implication was clear: Do it my way, or I'll see you at the funeral.

After their insensitive comments, I discontinued my relationship with both the surgeon and Jane. They were far too emotionally invested in their point of view. I was especially upset because they weren't honoring my choice, a choice that I didn't make lightly. I felt good about the decision; it was right for me. My radiologist was no fool and had consulted several major cancer centers around the country. Plus, he had dealt with anal cancer before, and I was pretty certain that the surgeon had not. I had confidence in the radiologist and confidence in my choice to go with his approach.

Months later, when I was doing forgiveness work, I discovered that I harbored a great deal of anger toward Jane. I had been seeing her for twelve years and was very fond of her. She was a passionate doctor, albeit test-crazy, and she was absolutely undone when my first diagnosis came up. I think she blamed herself for not catching the cancer sooner, since I had been going to her for years about the hemorrhoid. I wasn't mad at her for that, however. She was doing the best she could, and my cancer looked and acted no differently than other people's hemorrhoids. What enraged me was that she dismissed my choice and she heartlessly insinuated that I would probably die if I didn't get the biopsy.

It was way out of line, and I felt deeply betrayed. I wasn't able to shake my anger at her for many months, even after I decided I wanted and needed to forgive her. I prayed and prayed to forgive her, even though I felt rage every time I drove by her office. Eventually, grace stepped in, and one morning when I woke up, I was no longer angry with her. Sometimes, that's how forgiveness works. It's as though angels lift the burden from us.

You may also find that a doctor, nurse, or an alternative practitioner crosses a line that insults your integrity and personal authority. It can be very painful. Don't forget to forgive them, in addition to yourself. After all, your judgment of them is no less toxic than their judgment of you.

Turns out, the cancer did come back, but a biopsy of the external anal tissue would not have identified it. Had I gotten a biopsy, it would have created daily pain, and it would not have healed easily. I am grateful to this day that I made the choice I did. I'm grateful to myself for trusting the authority within that said no to the biopsy and yes to my radiologist's approach.

I believe we are given free will so we can discover the infinite power within that is the source of our own creative—and healing—genius. By knowing our own authority, we can better understand the Kingdom within.

Whether you choose conventional or alternative treatment, it is imperative that you be your own keeper, your own healer, your own patient, your own advocate, and your own authority—indeed, by the grace of God, your own greatest hope.

There ain't nothing from the outside can lick any of us.
MARGARET MITCHELL

RIC'S STORY

Man's mind, once it's stretched by a new idea, never regains its original dimensions.
OLIVER WENDELL HOLMES

Ric Johnson believes we don't know the difference between good luck and bad. That's saying something from a guy who, since 2002, has endured seventeen surgeries, five rounds of chemo, and a battalion of radiation, only to be told that the cancer was growing, and his doctors could do nothing more.

Ric, whose history is jammed with risk taking, didn't buy it. Although he wasn't happy with the news, he didn't give up. In fact, in 2008, he was the first cancer survivor to complete a deep-sea dive so challenging and complex that only a hundred people in the world have ever done it.

Ric's love of deep-sea diving and his attraction to high-stakes hobbies are a testament to his fearless passion for living life as an adventure. Prior to cancer, he owned a race-car business, rode dirt bikes, and did as much deep-sea diving as he could. That daring streak within him is part of what saved his life. But mostly he's diving today because of the "cocktail" provided by Dr. David Walker, an American now practicing in Mexico (see page 128).

That's the good luck part. Here's what many would consider the bad luck part: in 2002, when he was forty-three years old, Ric began experiencing pain in his lower gastrointestinal tract. He ignored it until blood appeared in his urine and stool. A day later, he was in the emergency room undergoing a CT scan. He knew he was in trouble when the nurse, who had been so cheerful before seeing the results of the film, approached him with obvious gloom. Shortly after, his wife and doctor arrived.

"We have some bad news for you," the doctor said. "There's a tumor the size of a grapefruit engulfing your colon."

If Ric agreed to chemo, radiation, and surgery, they said he would live for maybe six months. He jumped on the treatments.

Surgery removed the tumor, and ten days later, he began an intensive three-month chemo program. A month after starting the chemo, they were preparing him for radiation when they discovered that the cancer had penetrated his entire colon and migrated to his stomach. They told him, "There is no stopping it."

Ric underwent another round of chemo, administered through tubes that fed into a surgically implanted port. The drugs were injected into his body twenty-four hours a day, seven days a week, for twelve weeks.

"It was really powerful chemo," he told me. "I was very sick. I normally weigh 200 pounds, and I got down to 120. I lost some of my hair, and I was weak. They did another surgery and found that the cancer had gotten into my spleen and pancreas. They took out what they could and closed me up."

The surgery was followed by six more months of chemo and radiation, but the treatments did nothing to stop the cancer. The disease was now in the base of his heart and traveling into his esophagus.

Another surgery removed part of his stomach, the tail end of his pancreas, and his spleen. With cancer in his esophagus, and because of his diminished stomach, he could no longer take food through his mouth. He received nourishment through a feeding tube, a nightmare in and of itself. He remained thin and frail.

After Ric's fourth round of chemo, doctors performed another surgery, a partial Whipple, which removed a small section from his heart. After that, they believed the heart would be OK, but the esophagus was another story.

"The cancer was everywhere in my esophagus, so they did whatever surgeries they could through the throat, clipping here, cauterizing there. I went to universities and cancer centers and clinics all over the United States, including Mayo. They discovered more tumors, this time on my liver and kidney. It finally got to the point where they said there was no hope."

Meanwhile, Ric's personal life was crumbling. He and his wife had split up—a mutual decision following the advice of Ric's doctors that he move to a lower elevation and warmer climate than where he lived in Colorado. He went to Arizona; his wife stayed in Colorado. Meanwhile, because he was committed to paying 40 percent of the $2.5 million in medical bills, by the time he arrived in Arizona, he was penniless. He found a spot in the desert, set up a tent, and consumed canned nourishment that he put through the feeding tube. By then he was able to put some food through his mouth, esophagus, and stomach, but all he could afford was beans and hot dogs.

"The hardest part was that it devastated my family—especially my kids. My family was torn up. I was awful to everyone. It was very hard on me, and I wouldn't be telling the truth if I said I didn't get depressed.

"By the end of 2007, I was below 100 pounds and spiraling. The doctors wanted to perform more major surgeries. I just wanted to get some diving in. I thought it would be so much easier to run out of air rather than go through all that grief. Even though everyone was real generous and so many people had helped—my church back in Colorado, my friends, and my wife—it was hard. I wanted to go back to diving."

Then serendipity entered. A new friend from Spain, Itzi, suggested that Ric go to Mexico and look for a doctor who did alternative treatments. She even offered to go along and care for him.

"She said she'd sweat it out with me," Ric recalled with a chuckle. "We found a little duplex to rent, and through that transaction, we met a man whose father had major cancer and had gone to Dr. David Walker in San Carlos, Mexico. He suggested that we go see him as soon as possible. We did."

The Mayo Clinic sent Ric's medical records to Dr. Walker, after which he assessed the case. "He said I was unique because he had never met anyone who had been through so much and survived. But he also said that he hadn't had much luck with people who had been radiated as much as I had. People just didn't recover after all that radiation. I appreciated his honesty.

"He said it was up to me if I wanted to go through his treatment. I wanted to, but I didn't have any money. He told me we'd worry about the money later. Compared to the $2.5 million we had spent on treatment in the States, what he wanted was a drop in the bucket. I didn't have it, but he started me on treatment anyway. That was in January 2008."

The all-natural "cocktail" Dr. Walker uses was administered intravenously, but there were problems. Ric's veins were hard and tight due to the chemo and radiation. Because it was so difficult, Dr. Walker started slowly with only two treatments per week. He increased the treatments gradually until Ric received a cocktail every other day. Eventually, he grew strong enough to swallow the concoction so that it went directly to his digestive system.

At first, there was no change in his condition other than some long-awaited weight gain. Finally, in April 2008, Ric took a CEA test (a blood test that determines the level of cancer present in the body). A normal, cancer-free result measures at 2.5; smokers usually show up from 4.0 to 6.0. At his worst, Ric's results had showed a daunting 37, but the new numbers showed a welcome decline. He continued his work with Dr. Walker and grew steadily stronger.

That July, Ric visited the Mayo Clinic in Scottsdale, where they performed another CEA and CT scan. The results were stunning. "When the doctor came to report the test results, I couldn't tell if she was full of gloom or beside herself with excitement. Then she said,

'Ric, I don't have a clue what you're doing, but whatever you're doing, keep it up. The tumors on your kidney and liver have shrunk to half the size. They're dying. And your CEA is at 0.7. Anything under 1.0 is unheard of.'

"I didn't tell her about Mexico and Dr. Walker's cocktail because I wanted straight talk without any bias. Plus, I had to keep my insurance intact, and I thought it was better to keep what I was doing quiet."

In late July, Ric began deep sea-diving again. In August of 2008, he was given an opportunity to participate in a highly technical dive to the ocean floor to see the USS *Monitor*, a ship that battled the CSS *Virginia* and turned the tide of the Civil War.

"That battle was a pivotal point in the Civil War, and that 240-foot dive was a turning point in my life," Ric said, his smile apparent through the telephone wires. After his momentous dive, Ric began getting requests for interviews. People wanted to know more about him.

"There is life after cancer. I've devoted myself to helping others and to assisting Dr. Walker with the new hospital he's trying to start.

"As we speak, I am cancer free. I weigh 190 pounds, and my last CEA was 0.9. I won't even raise my eyebrows unless it goes over 4. I still take the cocktail once a month. I carry it with me everywhere I go—along with cans of food that were supposed to go through my feeding tube but that now I just drink down."

His recovery wasn't only physical. "While I was sick, Itzi saw me at my worst—my angriest, my meanest. She took off for Spain to visit family for four months, but we kept in close contact. While she was gone, I realized what she meant to me. She came back, we got together, and she never gave up on me. When there was no money, she paid. When I didn't want to deal with something, she was my rock. She's more honest and has more integrity than anyone I've ever known. She's the woman of my life.

"If it hadn't been for the cancer, I never would have met Itzi. I never would have met David. I wouldn't have made a difference in people's lives, wouldn't have devoted myself to humanity. That's what I mean when I say you don't know the difference between good luck and bad."

When I asked Ric if he had any idea why or how he got cancer, he said, "Cancer doesn't run in my family," and then took a moment before continuing. "I can't talk about what happened in my military life. It was classified. But I was around some very bad, toxic stuff.

"As far as my mind-set went, I had conflicts with my wife, and I regret them all. Yet I was still pretty happy in life. I survived crazy incidents in the military and playing with race cars and on dirt bikes. I had some serious things happen to me, but I always survived.

"I believe in God, and I believe that what's going to happen will happen. I've never been one to panic. Even through most of my cancer, I wasn't scared of dying. I've never looked at life as something I couldn't deal with. I never thought 'Woe is me,' even in the hardest times.

"Your mind-set is a big piece of healing. If you sit there and cry the blues, no offense, but you're putting the final nail in your coffin. You have to think positively, keep busy, don't let your mind dwell. It's easy to find yourself in the hole of depression because everything associated with cancer—the treatments and the attitudes—are as bad as the cancer itself.

"If you want to survive, you have to give it everything you can. If you think of gloom and doom, you'll lie down and die. I'm proud of the fact that I never let it get to that point."

Ric has about one-third of his stomach left, but due to the scar tissue, it will never heal. He can't sustain himself with food, so he continues to drink his feeding-tube supplement. Diet and exercise, Ric has learned, are vitally important to his overall well-being.

"Itzi feeds me healthy food. I lift weights, I swim a lot, and I'm very athletic. I'm healthier than I have been in years."

He's also happier. "There's a lot of good that's come out of this—a lot of self-realization and understanding of life and what it means to me. I know that the real treasure and wealth of life isn't about money or hot rods or fancy boats. It's what you do for humanity. I take off my shirt, and I see where a shark bit me. I see the many scars from surgeries. I see the port that attaches to the feeding tube, and I realize that I'm a wealthy person. It's made me stronger. I hug more. I express my love more. I resolve issues quietly. I'm proof to people that you can do it too."

As upbeat as he is, Ric feels that this experience also made him more cynical. "The American medical system doesn't want people to know about alternative medicine or curing cancer. There's no money in it. Dr. Walker's cocktail is all-natural, and the big drug companies can't make money off that. The money I've spent for Dr. Walker's treatment is pennies compared to the $2.5 million we threw at conventional treatment, to say nothing of the nightmares that that treatment caused. When you're in that system, you can feel like you're a prisoner, powerless and hopeless.

"My kind of cancer, mucinous adenocarcinoma, is considered one of the three deadliest kinds. Each year, the Mayo Clinic saves about fourteen people out of one hundred at stage 4 of this type of cancer. I'm sure that Dr. Walker's numbers are far better than that.

"But the other big part of healing is your brain. I've been in pain from my toes to my hair, but I used my brain as a tool to control myself, guide myself, and make things better. The brain never idles. You have to be tenacious. You have to look in the mirror and tell yourself, 'I'm not dying.' If you've got a mule in front of you and it won't move, then you kick it. Do anything to keep the motivation going."

Ric's son has moved in with him, and they're "best buddies." His daughter lives with his ex-wife in Colorado, and Ric claims that they're better friends now than during the years of cancer.

"I never give up. I continually smile and say, 'Damn, it's just another thing to deal with. That's life.'"
Just don't give up on trying to do what you really want to do. Where there is love and inspiration,
I don't think you can go wrong.

DAVID L. WALKER, PHD, NT, PM

Bio-Res-Med
Medical Arts Center

Never be bullied into silence. Never allow yourself to be made a victim. Accept no one's definition of your life; define yourself.
HARVEY FIERSTEIN

David L. Walker, PhD, is worth paying attention to. For starters, he's had cancer and was given one of those "get your affairs in order" prognoses. Lo and behold, today he's alive, thriving, and cancer free. He had been working as a biophysicist in the pharmaceutical industry, and ironically, he healed himself with natural remedies. Because he worked in the drug-making industry, he knows a little—scratch that, a *lot*—about what goes on inside the corridors of those multibillion-dollar companies, which is another reason to listen to him. And finally, the natural remedies that healed him were also created by him. He's now treating all kinds of "incurable" patients at the clinic he founded in San Carlos, Mexico. His story is compelling and fraught with the kind of drama that only high-stakes politics can craft.

In 1993, Dr. Walker entered the emergency room with excruciating pain and was told that his condition was likely appendicitis. The doctors performed their tests and then told him to call his family and notify them he was about to undergo surgery. When he awoke, his entire family was gathered around the bed, knowing that his grueling nine-hour surgery had nothing to do with appendicitis. He had advanced colon cancer, but no one told him this until four days after the surgery.

Once he caught on to the gravity of the situation, he knew it was dire. His oncologist said that if he did nothing, he would have a 10 percent chance of living. The good news was that he could try a new type of chemo and have a 40 percent chance of being alive for another two or three years. He agreed to the chemo.

After three surgeries and seven months of treatment, the cancer metastasized to his liver, abdomen, bladder intramuscular area, and testicles. "It was bad," he reports, but he wanted to quit the treatment because it was "killing me faster than the disease." This fact, combined with what he knew about the financial incentives of the medical system, made him turn away from conventional treatment.

"One doctor told me that if I quit working with him, he'd be out $350,000. Then there was the chemo. Since I worked in the business, I knew that the company who manufactured the chemo put ingredients in it that produced strong side effects. They also, of course, supplied a very expensive pill to mitigate the side effects. It's all about money, and I just wanted to get better."

Dr. Walker's doctors told him that he would certainly die without the treatments. That hit him hard. He had three young children who he was determined to see graduate from high school. His strength was that he was a cellular biologist and knew how cells worked. He decided to spend his final days experimenting with possible treatments. His education as a scientist and his desire to see his kids graduate mustered all the strength he needed to begin his work.

"There are five or six things that happen on a cellular level with the two hundred diseases we call cancer. I began combining things that I thought might impact the membrane penetration of the cancer cells. I knew membrane penetration was key, but I didn't know where to go from there. Eventually, I realized that I was approaching this in the same way I would as a pharmaceutical biologist—backward. That's when I stopped, pulled back, and began to see it differently, more simply. I just needed to find the elements that would be productive to the cancer-induced cell and its inability to accept medication or nutrients."

His studies continued, he had some breakthroughs, and he applied his custom-made concoctions to himself. Soon he began to feel better.

"That's all I could go on," he said. "I was petrified to go back into the medical system to get tested, so I just went on how I felt."

After eight months of drawing his own blood, conducting his own analyses, and ingesting his own natural remedies, Dr. Walker felt better at age forty-one than he had at age twenty-five.

Two years later, he decided to go back to his oncologist and let the mainstream medical system check him out. The tests came back clean. His doctor inferred that something was wrong and asked him to redo the tests. He did. Again the tests were clean. Not wanting to stir things up, Dr. Walker told his speechless oncologist that he had simply gone home after his last visit and prayed.

Dr. Walker doesn't emphasize praying as an integral part of healing from cancer, as he perceives most cancers are genetic in nature. That said, he does acknowledge that 80 percent of curing any disease is in the mind.

"We live in a society that kills people prematurely. Our minds and bodies are built to kill off negative influences. When you feel good, your mind produces endorphins, which can aid the remedies to penetrate the membranes. Endorphins produce a specific energy level and can, for example, convert bad food into better food. When your belief system is aligned with the action, the action will be supported by the whole mind. When the two are in sync, the body accepts the treatment without rejection. Whatever you have faith in will serve you."

Dr. Walker emphasized his point: "That applies to everything. When I was sick, I never thought of cancer and death as synonymous. I never saw it as what would kill me. My mind was made up. In the same way, if you are fully in support of pharmaceuticals, they will likely work in your favor. The backlash of that choice, however, is that the side effects are severe."

Dr. Walker knows a good bit about backlashes—as much from the side effects of drugs as from the politics of creating alternative cancer treatments.

After he healed himself, people started coming to him for help. He happily shared his newfound and effective remedies. As success stories began to spread through word of mouth and a website he built, more people came to him. He was gratefully having an 86 percent success rate with his clients.

"Mainstream treatment of chemo and radiation has about a 10 percent success rate over a ten-year period. I had an 86 percent success rate. You can't argue with that."

What the U.S. Food and Drug Administration (FDA) and the American Medical Association (AMA) did argue with, however, was that Dr. Walker didn't have a license to practice medicine. They proceeded to sue him for that and for his 14 percent mortality rate.

"I have been persecuted, prosecuted, sued, and harassed by state and federal government agencies," he says. "The rewards are there, however, for those of us who take our health care into our own hands."

Keeping an upbeat attitude while the suit was in progress was emotionally exhausting. The state of Washington, where he lived, hired a bevy of medical consultants to evaluate the charges, with the intention of rallying their support. In the end, all the consultants advised that the state drop the charges, which they did. But only six days later, the FDA, the Federal Trade Commission (FTC), and the Washington attorney general came after him, absconded with ten years' worth of paperwork he had kept while treating his cancer patients, and then sent the records to twelve different doctors for evaluation. The doctors again advised that the charges against Dr. Walker be dropped. The FDA and FTC complied, but the attorney general's office continued its suit, citing 320 counts of various offenses, in addition to Internet fraud.

After all was said and done, only two counts stood. One for claiming a 90 percent success rate on his website, and another for improper record keeping. Not a single doctor would testify that his protocol caused harm to anyone he treated. For those two offenses, they slapped Dr. Walker with an $800,000 fine, plus court costs and $400,000 in legal fees.

The judgment ruined him financially, and he was emotionally spent. His wife had worked a good job with retirement benefits, and they decided to move to Mexico where they could spend the rest of their lives wearing shorts and basking in the sun. Dr. Walker was finished with the cancer business; it had been too devastating. He would retire.

So he thought.

Success stories followed him across the border, and positive press spread the news about his noninvasive, natural remedies that had helped so many people. One such article was published in *Integrated Cancer and Oncology News (ICON)* magazine and *Positive Health* magazine,[2] both of which printed his home phone number in Mexico. The calls poured in, and that was the beginning of his so-called retirement.

"I had no intention of doing this, but I'll probably do it until the day I die," he said, referring to the work he has been doing since opening the Medical Arts Center and Bio-Res-Med in 2003 and offering Cellular Adaptive

Therapy. As of 2009, the clinic employed seven full-time medical doctors, oncologists, and acupuncturists, while also providing a fully equipped lab, hematoxology department, and high-tech diagnostic equipment for CT scans. His clinic is fully self-funded.

"My staff and I are firm believers in education. We'll give you all the education we can. By learning what cancer is and what we do to turn it around, you can make the most informed decision possible. I'm also working to educate other doctors about this therapy. I'm touring a lot, and I know what to say and how to say it."

He claimed that there are many doctors who want to help their patients with new approaches, but most of them still do only what's been approved by the FDA, which itself is deeply entangled with the pharmaceutical industry. "If the FDA wants," reported Walker, "they can come in and find a reason to close you down." For this reason, Dr. Walker has, at times, "accidentally" dropped his business card in the lobby of a hospital or clinic, especially where children are treated. Parents who pick up the cards call him and find new hope.

His own children are the inspiration for Dr. Walker's survival, and his love for children everywhere has moved him to construct a new hospital specifically for children with cancer. Much of the money to fund the hospital has come from donors grateful for their experiences of healing through his protocol. Still, he doesn't take all the credit.

"You have to have a reason to live, not just the will to. It has to be bigger than you. In my case, it was my kids. I had been active with them throughout their lives. I coached them in sports and never missed a recital. They were my life. The fear of them growing up without me was awful. And yes, I did see them graduate."

***

Postscript: When this book went to print, Dr. Walker informed me that he had just received a $338 million dollar grant from a private holding company in New York. According to Dr. Walker, the funds will "build my dream hospital and an international children's cancer treatment center in San Carlos. It will be a six hundred-bed facility and recreational park for handicapped and disabled kids, as well as a hotel for their parents."

Meanwhile, Dr. Walker's clinics are opening in Germany, France, Spain, and Bulgaria. He has also been invited by the Jordanian government to present his work to the Ministry of Health and start the medical training necessary for doctors to use his treatments on their cancer patients.

The Particulars

Where: Medical Arts Center, Bio-Res-Med, San Carlos, Mexico.

Who: David Walker, PhD, NT, PM, founder, with seven doctors on staff.

What to expect: You'll be asked to send diagnostic paperwork to the center. The medical board will decide whether or not to take your case.

"Certain types of cancer respond really well to our therapies while others don't," says Dr. Walker. "Still, we take plenty of patients that other centers turn down. It's important to remember that we cannot reverse damage that's been done by other treatments; rather, we stop the growth so that there is no more damage."

Once you are at the center, doctors establish your baseline by performing their own diagnostics through CTs and MRIs, blood panels, the history of previous treatments, medicines and supplements, and so forth. Everything else is rooted in monitoring progress.

Every patient is given a tailor-made healing protocol. Even people with the same cancers have different treatments based on their unique chemistry. All the products they use are natural and derived from plants, enzymes, Indian elementals, and so on. The therapy may be administered orally, intravenously, topically, or through micronutrients. Their objective is to increase the alkalinity and oxygenation within the body, at which time the tumor can no longer survive.

Once the tumor markers are down, you can go home, although you may visit the clinic for periodic treatment for years. Dr. Walker still self-administers his healing protocol for thirty days once a year.

Typical routine: Patients are treated every other day with two sessions per day. They spend about two hours at the clinic. The rest of the time is free. The town is inexpensive and beautiful.

Where to stay: The clinic is located in a resortlike setting with nine small apartments, a swimming pool, and lovely surroundings. At the time of our interview, the lease on the facility was almost up, and they were possibly going to move into another building that does not have housing accommodations. The new building is close to an affordable resort where patients can stay. People with lengthier stays often rent apartments close to the center; some stay with San Carlos residents, and many stay in hotels.

Cost: The treatments range from $1,500 (for some skin cancers) to $86,000 for the worst cases with multiple problems. An average person spends $30,000 and stays between six to ten weeks. More specifically, average costs are about $3,700 per week of therapy. Everyone goes home with six months' worth of remedies.

Who goes: Most of the clientele is European, although there are some Americans and Canadians. The clinic treats all kinds of cancer, but has the best success with breast and skin cancers.

Words of wisdom: Dr. Walker believes strongly in self-education.

"The key to any successful therapy is education. Find out what's available and determine what you can believe in and support. I can share with you what I know, but what you do with it is your business. The greatest thing you can do for yourself is self-education, rather than thinking that mainstream treatment is all you have and all that there is. That's just not true."

Contact Information:

Offices & Laboratorios
Hacienda Plaza
Lote 264 Sector El Creston

San Carlos, Sonora, 85506
Mexico

From outside Mexico phone:
011-52-622-226-1977
Fax: 011-52-622-226-1987
bioresmed.com
bioresmedclinic.com

Only a man who knows what it is like to be defeated can reach down to the bottom of his soul and come up with the extra ounce of power it takes to win when the match is even.
MUHAMMAD ALI

CHAPTER 5

Energy

What the caterpillar calls the end of the world the master calls a butterfly.
RICHARD BACH

I still marvel at the concept that everything is energy. The first time I heard the idea, I couldn't quite grasp that I am nothing more than antimatter. I'm a material girl, after all. I mean, I have a body, and it's very real. I know that especially when I experience extreme pain or pleasure. I drive a car, and it's solid as steel, right? It even has safety devices like air bags, so if I'm in a collision, this very real body of mine won't get battered. Then, of course, I live in a house that is strong enough to keep out fits of stormy weather. So what's all this business that everything is nothing but energy?

Experts say it's pretty simple. Everything on our planet, including our bodies, cars, homes, all that accumulated stuff, and everything both seen and unseen, reduces down to particles of energy. Dense energy is represented through physical forms like our bodies, rocks, trees, and so on. Likewise, nonphysical energy is represented through air, light, thoughts, emotions, and spirit. People reflect both physical and nonphysical energy. When you really and truly absorb this concept, then you accept that cancer is energy, too.

Here's how I think it plays out: Our physical bodies are cauldrons of nonphysical energy. Our minds are the opening through which nonphysical energy passes. The flow doesn't stop at the site of the brain. It pours down into our bodies, feeding them with the nature of our thoughts and emotions—the nonphysical stuff.

Thoughts and emotions have an innate frequency or vibrational tone, which is absorbed throughout our bodies. There isn't just a tiny opening between our minds and our bodies that secretes a slight bit of currency from one arena to the next, thus creating the famous "mind-body connection." (That term always feels to me like it is shortchanging a magnificent marriage.) Rather, there is a continuous surge of messages circulating between the physical body and the nonphysical mind.

In short, the brain receives physical needs and sensations from the body, while the body captures the quality of the frequency within the mind. Every organ within us, every fiber, cell, molecule, bone, and fluid—everything that makes up our organic chemistry—is party to the energy either generated in or filtered through the mind. Our minds and bodies make up a single—albeit complex—unit made up of nonphysical energy and biological matter constantly at play with each other.

Most of us believe that our thoughts are isolated and heard only by the perceiver within (which can include God). Our minds are the most private place we occupy. Even the people closest to us, the ones we love and exchange intimacies with, can never know the breadth and depth of the thoughts and feelings we entertain, dodge, fear, indulge in, aspire to, or harbor. Our minds, however, are not isolated; they are married to our bodies, the mouthpiece of our consciousness. Our bodies can speak volumes, not only about lifestyle and eating habits, but also about what's stored in the most secret and remote corners of our consciousness.

No one but the self really knows what goes on inside the mind, but the body can decode the energetic tone and reveal it through physical imbalances and illness. It's easy to recognize this dynamic. When we worry, we can't sleep, and we may develop headaches or, eventually, an ulcer. Likewise, when we feel love and joy, there's a noticeable lilt in our step; we enjoy unlimited energy, and eventually, we experience fewer and fewer physical discomforts. Sometimes, they disappear completely.

Our bodies enable us to know what's being conjured in our minds. How would we know we were sad if we didn't experience a heaviness in our arms and legs? How would we know we were afraid if the pit of our stomach didn't tighten? How would we know the depth of our love if we didn't feel it in every cell of the body? Our bodies are the greatest gauges for informing us about ourselves.

The emotional quality (or vibration) in which we dwell is the product of feelings and thoughts. A feeling doesn't happen on its own. It's the physical expression of thought. Yet our thoughts are lightning fast, and often they knock around in our subconscious mind—a place we can't hear very well. This means that we often aren't even aware of the thoughts that we embrace or the vibration we carry. But our bodies tell it all.

It's important to pay attention to how we feel. Our thoughts will evade us, but our feelings are easy to identify. If we feel bad and allow those bad feelings to persist, they will probably settle into the body, which will soon enough articulate those thoughts and feelings through illness or disease.

This isn't to say that we can never again think a thought that makes us feel bad. That's part of being human. The question is, how often or how long do we entertain those thoughts? Some people get a thrill out of feeling bad. Many are addicted to drama. Look at the movies, video games, and television shows that add to a mounting mistrust of others. It's essential to pay attention to how we feed the fears we possess. It's important to discern whether we're protecting our fears because we believe they will somehow protect us from the forces "out there." It's much easier to justify fear than to release it, especially if we feel like it's a necessary and important armor in a world gone mad.

Fear delights in all the things that separate us from others and from ourselves. It uses blame, helplessness, powerlessness, anger, resentment, judgment, cruelty, guilt, shame, and all the other "negative" emotions to keep itself alive. These feelings are honest indications that the thoughts we are thinking, whether we're aware of them or not, are not serving our higher purpose.

Thankfully, thoughts are fluid, and we can change them. Yet since thoughts are so slippery, and more often than not doggedly habitual, it's easier simply to work on changing our feelings. When we commit to focusing on things that make us feel better, we elevate the energetic tone within.

This is simple, but not necessarily easy, especially when we believe that our negative thoughts and feelings are justified. (And who doesn't?) Still, the payoff for committing to releasing negative thoughts and giving ourselves to positive ones is huge.

Here's an example of how my husband, Ed, ultimately transcended a very old habit of acting out his negative feelings and why he was glad he did. One sunny day, he was driving our new, pretty, red Prius when a guy in a big 4x4 pulled out in front of him. Ed laid on the horn, after which the guy in the 4x4 slammed on the brakes. Ed was happy to pass him (with a few hand gestures) and be done with the interaction, but within seconds the 4x4 was tailgating him. The driver was giving him the finger and visibly ranting. A mile later and a little spooked, Ed decided to take a turn to get this guy off his tail. The driver followed, however, making the situation even more tense. Ed then pulled a U-turn so he could go back to the main road. The

4x4 followed, and instead of pulling up behind Ed, the driver aimed for the side of our perfect little Prius, stepped on the gas, and rammed into the car.

By then, Ed was scared. Was this guy carrying a gun? How far would he go? Dazed, he sat in the car grappling with the fact that this maniac had just rammed our cute little baby with his mammoth SUV.

Seconds later, the driver was headed for Ed's door. Instinctively, Ed jumped out of the car ready to defend himself and was amazed when he saw the driver pleading for his forgiveness, begging Ed not to call the police. Filled with regret, he said that his wife had just left him and that he had snapped. He would do whatever was necessary to pay for the repairs. Ed's heart opened up, and he agreed to handle the damages outside of the legal system.

Long story short, the driver was in the insurance business and knew exactly how to bypass his responsibility to pay for repairs. He had conned Ed with his feigned remorse, and although Ed did what he could to recover the money, the local district attorney told Ed that since he hadn't called the cops, he had little chance of winning in court.

Ed was livid. Not only had this guy rammed our most favorite car ever, he deceived Ed and left us with the bill. Anyone can understand the anger, resentment, feelings of powerlessness, and fury my sleepless husband experienced.

On top of all that, Ed doesn't sit still for disrespect. His big button is all about being disrespected, and if he feels that he's been dissed, the warrior in him surfaces with thick armor and plenty of ammo. He pulls out all the stops.

He oozed with anger and rage. He obsessed. He spent hours talking to attorneys and telling the story repeatedly to aghast friends. He thought he could take the man to court, and even though he hadn't called the cops, a jury would surely empathize with him and make things right. He knew where the guy lived and worked. He spent hours fantasizing the taste of sweet revenge.

Before all this could make Ed sick, however, he caught himself. He's a fighter by nature, but Ed knew that going after this guy would require more time and energy than it was worth. More importantly, by engaging in a tenuous legal battle, he would keep alive the intensely negative feelings he had been drowning in since the incident. In essence, it was he, Ed, who was suffering because of these feelings.

Consequently, after months of upset, Ed decided to let it go. I had been hoping for that, but I know my husband and didn't expect it. It took diligence and practice, but eventually he didn't think about the incident anymore, didn't well up with ideas of retaliation, didn't even keep an eye out for that fateful 4x4. He let it go, and with that, he broke a lifelong pattern of allowing spiteful energies to determine the quality of his life. It freed him to create new energetic patterns that have given him (and us) more peace. It strengthened him in ways he's still enjoying. It was one of the greatest leaps in his life.

Four years later, we learned that the driver of the 4x4 was killed in an automobile accident. We never learned the circumstances of the crash, but both Ed and I were surprised at how it affected us. This guy had played an instrumental role in Ed's evolution of consciousness. We're not the judges of why this tragedy occurred, but in the context of our lives, it was poignant. We were both saddened that he was killed.

It was true for Ed, and it is true for all of us: upon deciding to release our anger and committing to feeling good, our bodies receive messages that are generative and healing. Soon enough, the vibrational tone is manifested physically.

People have a hard time with this concept because they are accustomed to thinking that things happen randomly and believing that we live in a world where we are all victims of genes, karma, or circumstance. Certainly these are influential, but I believe that more often than not, we create our emotional and physical imbalances because of where we dwell energetically. Sometimes we dwell in these places out of habit; sometimes we do so because we don't adequately express our emotions, and they get locked up in our cells.

I've always been an upbeat person. After my first diagnosis, it was hard for me to buy into the idea that my vibration created the disease. People who know and love me consider me to be positive and optimistic, and they often said, "You are the most positive person I know. How could cancer be a product of your thoughts? It doesn't make any sense."

At first, it didn't make sense to me either, but when I really and truly monitored my feelings and camped out in the wilderness of my mind—a place that only I can go—I began to recognize some discreet but ubiquitous demons. I had lived with them my entire life, and so I thought they were normal. The king of them all, and the one who fathered the lesser ones, has always been fear.

I've done a lot of work to release myself from fear, and I've come a long way. Now that my body is relieved of much of it, I feel lighter, freer, more relaxed, and far more energized. It's stunning to me now that I'd thought being clenched in my gut, stiff in my shoulders, and always on alert was simply a normal way of being. I believe my cancer was, in part, a result of a low energetic tone I harbored inside myself. I believe much of my healing came about by exchanging those low frequencies for higher ones.

On the one hand, by taking an honest inventory of our inner environment, we can determine if our thoughts yield feelings of depression, anger, sadness, or any other outcroppings of fear. If so, cancer may well be the clarion call for a new mind-set. When we consider that there are millions of people on antidepressants, millions more who cradle no excitement for life, and still more millions who numb their anguish with addictions to drugs, alcohol, comfort food, pornography, sex, or video games, it's no wonder that cancer affects nearly half of our population. It's easy to recognize that our bodies are crying out on behalf of our souls.

On the other hand, when we do whatever's necessary to foster feelings of joy, contentment, appreciation, playfulness, tenderness, compassion, generosity, and love for others and ourselves, we create the best possible environment, both internally and externally, for cancer to resolve itself.

If you honestly believe that your vibration dwells in the attributes of love, and you've still contracted cancer, it could be due to an external environmental toxin, an inherited gene gone bad, or an enigmatic spiritual necessity. The mystery can be confounding, but trusting the process, the reason, the meaning, is essential. Hating what is and blaming others or yourself only exacerbate the intensity of the experience and feelings of hopelessness. Allowing yourself to grow into whatever happens, whatever will be, without dwelling in rage or regret is a great act of courage and love that results in peace. May we all be blessed with that kind of peace when we cross from this world to the next.

We either make ourselves miserable or we make ourselves strong. The amount of work is the same.
CARLOS CASTANEDA

JEFF'S STORY

Ruin and recovery are both from within.
EPICTETUS

Jeff was a serious athlete, and in 1988, he had just completed a grueling day of cross-country skiing when he felt a pain in his groin.

"It was a rough ski, very icy, and I figured I had stretched something. After a few days, it was still hurting, so I went to a doctor. He told me I was working out too hard and to just take some aspirin, and I'd be fine. That was in February."

The aspirin didn't help. Over the next five months, Jeff visited three doctors, but none were able to get to the root of the problem. Finally, he went to a physical therapist specializing in sports injuries. After walking from one side of the room to the other, the PT said, "You've got something wrong with your pelvis. The symptoms say it's cracked. Let's get some X-rays."

The pictures revealed irregularities on the right side of his pelvic socket. "About two-thirds of it looked like cardboard," Jeff recalled. "The PT told me I needed a biopsy, but it never occurred to me that it might be cancer."

It was. In mid-August, Jeff was shocked with the news that he had an unusual type of multiple myeloma, a blood-and-bone marrow cancer that results in tumors cropping up all over the body. It typically shows up first in the longer bones of ribs, legs, and arms. Uncharacteristically, his started in the groin and pelvis.

Jeff's oncologist believed that five weeks of radiation would help, but during treatments, Jeff was knocked flat. "They had no way to radiate me without getting some of my internal organs. My intestines were burned from the inside out. The pain was horrible. I couldn't eat. I got down to 127 pounds. It was very hard."

The cancer was spreading fast. Prior to the radiation, it had moved into his thigh and traveled down to his knee.

Consequently, he was already weak. But on October 10, ten days after the radiation treatments ended, Jeff was concerned; though he was no longer getting treatment, the effects of the radiation were continuing. "I told my doctor that I'd be in a wheelchair pretty soon if it didn't stop. I was getting weaker and weaker, losing the feeling in my legs and having tingling in my arms. They did a spinal tap and discovered that the cancer had spread into the spinal fluid."

The next stop was the Mayo Clinic. They retested Jeff, only to find that his condition had worsened. There was talk of a bone-marrow transplant, but the final decision was to treat him with chemotherapy applied directly into the spine.

"That type of treatment hadn't been done much, so the doctors weren't sure if it would work," Jeff said. "And if it did work, I'd probably end up paralyzed."

He refused the chemo.

"That's when they told me that I'd better get my affairs in order because I had two, maybe three months left.

"The truth is, I wasn't afraid of dying. When I was eleven years old, I got run over by a tractor. The doctors told my parents I had been killed. I had an out-of-body experience and saw myself under that tractor. Having that experience changed the way I looked at life. I was really OK with dying.

"I thought a little about getting from here to there, but I wasn't even sad about leaving loved ones behind. I'm pragmatic. I was married at the time and had a big life insurance policy. I figured my wife would be fine."

Upon returning home, Jeff was indeed wheelchair bound, although he could "shuffle around with a cane" if necessary. Since he had been in such good shape prior to the cancer, being so weak—and in a wheelchair—was deeply disturbing. Added to that was the psychological distress. "The doctors were afraid to give me hope about anything. I knew that couldn't be good for me, but I moped around for a few weeks anyway. Finally, I got up and decided to work out. I walked to the mailbox. I did a push-up. I went back to the PT and asked him to put me on a machine that would exercise my leg muscles. Then I went for my last haircut."

During the haircut, his stylist asked Jeff what he was doing about his situation. When Jeff had no response, she asked, "Are you open to seeing a spiritualist?"

"I had been raised on religion, and it had done nothing for me. But I didn't know what a spiritualist was, and yes, I was open to anything.

"His name was Ben, and he lived on a mesa. I was thirty-seven years old at the time, and Ben was seventy. Yet he looked younger than I did. He told me about himself and asked what he could do for me.

"'They tell me I'm going to die,' I said. 'I thought I'd ask you for suggestions.'

"He looked at me and simply said, 'You go home and decide if they can tell you that you're going to die. If you determine that the answer is no, then come back and see me.'

"After about a week, I determined that the answer was no, *no one else can tell you when you're going to die.*

So I went back to him, and he taught me how to meditate. He did guided meditation with me, also known as creative visualization. Every day I went to Ben's for an hour or two. He never took money. He told me that I needed to go into my spine and clean it up myself. He said, 'You've got to be able to go outside your body and then come back into the parts that need work. You can go there, to the part that needs work, and make the changes.'

"I took it from there. What I ended up doing was envisioning my spine as a big hallway. I'd walk through a door and be in this big, long hallway full of all kinds of horrible-looking liquid and nasty-looking fish, as if I were underwater. They were clinging to the sides of the hallway. I first took nets and caught the fish. I'd do this for about thirty minutes, three or four times a day. Over time, I could tell there was a difference, and there were fewer and fewer fish.

"Eventually in these meditations, two maids showed up. They were even in maid's outfits and everything. I wasn't coached on this; they just showed up, and they had all kinds of cleaning tools. They didn't say anything to me; they just went to work cleaning the hallway. In about another week, the liquid was all cleaned up."

Jeff had been going to his doctor's office once a week so the doctor could monitor the progress of the cancer. At this point, the doctor took a test and told Jeff that they were having lab problems and would have to take another test. Jeff said he knew the test was clean, but the doctor replied that such a thing couldn't happen. A second test came back clean—no cancer. The doctor was perplexed and had no clue what had happened. Jeff said, "He gave no credence to anything outside of the medical profession. Of course, I told him nothing about the meditations." Soon Jeff's legs began to function again. "The last day I went through a meditation, the hallway—my spine—was completely clean. Then a spirit showed up. He had a staff, which he set down, and then he crossed his arms. He was basically telling me I was good to go.

"Even after that, I'd have some fears. I'd wake up in a cold sweat, for example. But then I'd meditate, and the spirit would come to me. I'd feel OK, and then I'd sleep like a puppy."

It was only six weeks from the time Jeff was told to get his affairs in order to the time he was found to be cancer free. He regained 70 percent of his thighs and 80 percent of his legs. Now, more than twenty years later, Jeff has regained his life as an athlete.

Given that he doesn't subscribe to religion, I asked him where he got the strength to believe in his healing. "I've asked myself that a lot," he said contemplatively. "I think I was born with it. I've always known that if I am going to be successful, I have to *believe* in it. I have to believe I am going to succeed and *know* that about myself.

"I use tennis as a metaphor. My goal isn't to win, but to play as well as I can. That's the way I measure myself. When I was faced with dying, I wanted to make sure that if there were anything I could do to change it, I would. If I couldn't, at least I'd give it my best shot so that I could die peacefully."

Jeff then talked about the peace he lives with now. "Once I whipped it, cancer was probably the best thing that ever happened to me. There's something to be said for spending time counting down the minutes. I remember sitting in the living room, watching the leaves blow off the trees and thinking that it was my last autumn. Then there was the time I was sitting in the Minneapolis airport, watching people walk down the concourse and laughing, and in my mind I'd say, 'The only difference between us is that I know when I'm going to die, and they don't.'"

Ben's influence was clearly instrumental in Jeff's healing. "Ben guided me through all this. He taught me that I wasn't separate from my body. I had been abusing my body before. I worked out too hard and put too much stress on it. I was a runner and had a three-mile course I'd laid out. I would go out and run it three times a week. I wanted to run it in less than twenty-one minutes. If I failed, my punishment was to push myself even harder. Ben changed that.

"Plus, Ben got me in touch with something else. He said, 'Every day, every second, your body is recreating itself on a cellular level. That cell, at some point, determines whether it's going to be a good cell or a bad cell. You just need to coach that cell into being a good cell.'

"That makes so much sense to me. I remember reading about statistics at the Mayo Clinic, and I thought, 'No. You either have cancer 100 percent, or you don't have it 100 percent.' Ben's comments really backed that up. He helped me find my lifeline. He helped me feel very secure that there is something better than religion out there for me."

I asked Jeff if he thought that lifeline would have come to him without Ben's help. "I'd hate to have to handicap that," he said. "When I went to Ben, I was open-minded. I wasn't a skeptic. I'm always open to something that feels good to me. The question is, would I have had the energy to explore it on my own? I don't know."

When asked what his lifeline is, he replied, "My spirit. That spirit with the staff, that's my spirit—my lifeline."

Jeff's story is truly remarkable, but over these past two decades, he's kept it largely to himself. "I determined early on that I wasn't going to communicate what I was feeling and thinking. Once I finally got to the point where I could take care of myself, I didn't want to carry all the doubters with me.

"This was an intense time when I had to go inside myself. I wasn't very communicative. I didn't have as much appreciation for the fear my wife was having. In fact, by the time I was healed, I knew I would stay healthy. But she could never give herself to believing that. Her fear was something that I had to cope with, but she couldn't resolve it. Eventually, we split up.

"The only other people I shared this with were my parents. My mother wanted me to talk to a friend who'd been diagnosed, but I couldn't do it. I'm comfortable with what I've got, but as soon as others start hanging on me, I'm afraid I could lose us both. I've got a lifeline that works for me, and others have to find the lifeline that works for them."

When asked if he believes there was an emotional component that gave him the cancer, Jeff replied, "My intellect would say yes, there was, but I don't know what it was. What I do know is that I gave it to myself because I didn't listen to my body. It gave me hints and finally hit me with a club."

Jeff's final advice was as straightforward as his own experience: "I'm not a go-over-the-edge kind of guy, but this whole thing changed my perspective. Cancer happens on the cellular level. Those are *your* cells. It's a simple deal: just get them to make the right choice. It's your body. If you want to move your thumb, you move your thumb. If you want to change your cells, you can do that, too."

The thing always happens that you really believe in; and the belief in a thing makes it happen.
FRANK LLOYD WRIGHT

BRUCE LIPTON, PHD

Epigenetics
Author of *The Biology of Belief:*
Unleashing the Power of Consciousness,
Matter, and Miracles

Be not afraid of life. Believe that life is
worth living, and your belief will help
create the fact.
WILLIAM JAMES

Dr. Bruce Lipton is a diehard scientist. He's devoted his life to understanding human biology and behavior. He received his PhD from the University of Virginia at Charlottesville, and then went on to the University of Wisconsin School of Medicine, where he was an associate professor of anatomy.

With his traditional track record, why do some people see him as controversial? Why did he step down from teaching medical students and strike out on a career path few had traveled? Simply put, Dr. Lipton has discovered that things aren't what they seem to be. Nor are they what he was teaching in med school or what we've been told to believe.

"Our health is not controlled by genetics," he told me in his characteristically upbeat and excited manner. "Conventional medicine is operating from an archaic view that we're controlled by genes. This misunderstands the nature of how biology works."

Medical professionals from around the globe may curl their lips and snarl, but Dr. Lipton's research—and the empirical evidence of colleagues—is forcing the issue enough so that changes in medical-school curriculums are currently underway.

But let's back up for a moment and sit through a blessedly unscientific explanation of Lipton's mind-expanding logic and what is known as epigenetics, "the study of inherited changes in phenotype (appearance) or gene expression caused by mechanisms other than changes in the underlying DNA sequence."

"Medicine does miracles," he said, "but it's limited to trauma. The AMA protocol is to regard our physical body like a machine, in the same way that an auto mechanic regards a car. When the parts break, you replace them—a transplant, synthetic joints, and so on—and those are medical miracles.

"The problem is that while they have an understanding that the mechanism isn't working, they're blaming the vehicle for what went wrong. They believe that the vehicle, in this case our bodies, is controlled by genes.

"But guess what? They don't take into consideration that there's actually a *driver* in that car. The new science, epigenetics, reveals that the vehicles—or the genes—aren't responsible for the breakdown. It's the driver."

In essence, if you don't know how to drive, you're going to mess up the vehicle. In the simplest translation, we can agree that lifestyle is the key to taking care of ourselves. Think well, eat well, and exercise, and your body won't break down and need new parts.

Dr. Lipton refers to the work of Dr. Dean Ornish to extrapolate. "Dr. Ornish has taken conventional cardiovascular patients, provided them with important lifestyle insights (better diet, stress-reduction techniques, and so on), and without drugs, the cardiovascular disease was resolved. Ornish relayed that if he'd gotten the same results with a drug, every doctor would be prescribing it."

That's fine and dandy for people with heart disease, diabetes, or obesity, but what about cancer? Even the strictest lifestyle changes don't cure cancer in everyone. What about genetic predispositions to getting the disease? "It used to be that we thought a mutant gene caused cancer," Lipton admitted, "but with epigenetics, all of that has changed."

Then he explained how his research revealed the science of epigenetics. "I placed one stem cell into a culture dish, and it divided every ten hours. After two weeks, there were thousands of cells in the dish, and they were all genetically identical, having been derived from the same parent cell. I divided the cell population and inoculated them in three different culture dishes.

"Next, I manipulated the culture medium—the cell's equivalent of the environment—in each dish. In one dish, the cells became bone, in another, muscle, and in the last dish, fat. This demonstrated that the genes didn't determine the fate of the cells because they all had the exact same genes. The environment determined the fate of the cells, not the genetic pattern. So if cells are in a healthy environment, they are healthy. If they're in an unhealthy environment, they get sick."

Dr. Lipton then took this a step further, which brings us back to the cancer question. "Here's the connection: With fifty trillion cells in your body, the human body is the equivalent of a skin-covered petri dish. Moving your body from one environment to another alters the composition of the 'culture medium,' the blood. The chemistry of the body's culture medium determines the nature of the cell's environment within you. The blood's chemistry is largely impacted by the chemicals emitted from your brain. Brain chemistry adjusts the composition of the blood based upon your perceptions of life. So this means that your perception of any given thing, at any given moment, can influence the brain chemistry, which, in turn, affects the environment where your cells reside and controls their fate. In other words, your thoughts and perceptions have a direct and overwhelmingly significant effect on cells."

This echoes, from a highly scientific point of view, what the intuitive and spiritual healers have been advocating for years: your mind can and does contribute to both the cause and healing of whatever ails you—including cancer.

Other than the mind, two other factors impact the fate of cells, according to Dr. Lipton: toxins and trauma. All three factors have been associated with the onset of cancer.

With this body of knowledge comes promising news. According to Dr. Lipton, gene activity can change on a daily basis. If the perception in your mind is reflected in the chemistry of your body, and if your nervous system reads and interprets the environment and then controls the blood's chemistry, then you can literally change the fate of your cells by altering your thoughts. In fact, Dr. Lipton's research illustrates that by changing your perception, your mind can alter the activity of your genes and create over thirty thousand variations of products from each gene. He gives more detail by saying that the gene programs are contained within the nucleus of the cell, and you can rewrite those genetic programs through changing your blood chemistry.

In the simplest terms, this means that we need to change the way we think if we are to heal cancer. "The function of the mind is to create coherence between our beliefs and the reality we experience," Dr. Lipton said. "What that means is that your mind will adjust the body's biology and behavior to fit with your beliefs. If you've been told you'll die in six months and your mind believes it, you most likely will die in six months. That's called the nocebo effect, the result of a negative thought, which is the opposite of the placebo effect, where healing *is* mediated by a positive thought."

That dynamic points to a three-party system: there's the part of you that swears it doesn't want to die (the conscious mind), trumped by the part that believes you will (the doctor's prognosis mediated by the subconscious mind), which then throws into gear the chemical reaction (mediated by the brain's chemistry) to make sure the body conforms to the dominant belief. (Neuroscience has recognized that the subconscious controls 95 percent of our lives.)

Now what about the part that doesn't want to die—the conscious mind? Isn't it impacting the body's chemistry as well? Dr. Lipton said that it comes down to how the subconscious mind, which contains our deepest beliefs, has been programmed. It is these beliefs that ultimately cast the deciding vote.

"It's a complex situation," said Dr. Lipton. People have been programmed to believe that they're victims and that they have no control. We're programmed from the start with our mother and father's beliefs. So, for instance, when we got sick, we were told by our parents that we had to go to the doctor because the doctor is the authority concerning our health. We all got the message throughout childhood that doctors were the authority on health and that we were victims of bodily forces beyond our ability to control. The joke, however, is that people often get better while on the way to the doctor. That's when the innate ability for self-healing kicks in, another example of the placebo effect.

"Jesuits used to say, 'Give me a child until age six or seven, and he'll be with the church for the rest of his life.' They knew that our subconscious minds are programmed through the experiences we have in the first six years of our lives.

"Since the subconscious programs operate outside the range of consciousness, we don't experience ourselves playing out these behaviors. Therefore, we don't even see ourselves sabotaging our own lives, and as a result, we don't take responsibility for the lives we lead. We see ourselves as victims of forces outside of our control. It's hard to own what we've done our whole lives. So we perceive ourselves as victims, and we believe that genes are in control."

I understand how reclaiming our power can help us heal—that doing so is, in fact, necessary for us to truly heal. Yet too many positive thinkers know that thinking good thoughts—and reciting affirmations for hours on end—doesn't always bring about the results that feel-good books promise.

Dr. Lipton didn't argue this point, because positive thoughts come from the conscious mind, while contradictory negative thoughts are usually programmed in the more powerful subconscious mind.

"The major problem is that people are aware of their conscious beliefs and behaviors, but not of subconscious beliefs and behaviors. Most people don't even acknowledge that their subconscious mind is at play, when the fact is that the subconscious mind is a million times more powerful than the conscious mind and that we operate 95 to 99 percent of our lives from subconscious programs.

"Your subconscious beliefs are working either for you or against you, but the truth is that you are not controlling your life, because your subconscious mind supersedes all conscious control. So when you are trying to heal from a conscious level—citing affirmations and telling yourself you're healthy—there may be an invisible subconscious program that's sabotaging you."

The power of the subconscious mind is elegantly revealed in people expressing multiple personalities. While occupying the mind-set of one personality, the individual may be severely allergic to strawberries. Then, in experiencing the mind-set of another personality, he or she eats them without consequence.

Even though the influence of our subconscious is interesting, on the face of it, this is not great news for those of us who are doing all we can to heal with our conscious minds. If health is largely determined by subconscious beliefs I'm not even aware of, then I'm brought right back to the original programming: I'm a victim with no control!

Dr. Lipton went on: "I used to say, 'You are personally responsible for everything in your life,' but people would look at me as if I'd slapped them. Now I say, 'Once you become aware of the fact that invisible programs from the subconscious mind are running your life, then you are responsible for it.'

"Becoming aware means accessing the behavioral programs in your unconscious mind so that you can change the underlying limiting or self-sabotaging thoughts that don't serve you. It's easy to figure out the nature of your subconscious programs. Just take a look at the character of your life. It's a printout of your subconscious programs. The things you're having trouble with are because of that programming."

Freeing Emotions and Anxiety

After learning about the role that the subconscious mind can have on health, I went on a hunt to learn more. I came upon Dr. Peter Lambrou and Dr. George Pratt's book, *Instant Emotional Healing: Acupressure for the Emotions.* It is an exciting book that teaches readers how to use the Emotional Self-Management (ESM) technique to change subconscious beliefs. Like some other energy treatments, it employs tapping on specific acupuncture points to get the job done.[1]

I called Dr. Lambrou, and he agreed to contribute his insights into the relationship between cancer and the subconscious mind.

***

"The connection between emotions, stress, and cancer is being recognized and validated with more clinical research each year. In my own practice, I've worked with several cancer survivors who have committed themselves to managing their stress and eliminating emotional residue from their past. This brief case example captures the essence of what I'm saying.

"Vickie was diagnosed with cancer and had two surgeries and other treatments. Three years ago, she came to me for psychological help to rid herself of anger and resentment toward her father for his distance and aloofness during her childhood, and toward her mother for being critical and demanding in those years. These unresolved emotions had been bothering her for nearly four decades, and she firmly believed they contributed to her developing ovarian cancer.

"We used the procedures of Emotional Self-Management described in *Instant Emotional Healing* to neutralize those old toxic emotions and to help her better manage her stress and anxiety in more current matters, such as her biannual CT scans.

"In Vickie's words: 'It's not so much the CT scan itself that's so stressful; it's waiting for the results. Nearly a week after the scan, I meet with my doctor, who's a good guy, and he explains each scan result in details that don't get to the real point until the very end. Waiting that thirty minutes can seem like half a day. With the 'tapping' that's used in Emotional Self-Management, I can get calm and patient and even expect good results while I listen.'

"The methods of the mind-body therapies work quickly and target specific emotional problems that persist and don't appear affected by ordinary 'talk therapy' or other methods.

"I believe that providing patients with self-applied techniques for managing their emotions enables them to develop a great sense of empowerment. So many aspects of life with cancer feel outside of our control, and this empowerment may well be a curative element that extends quality and length of life. In fact, such a sense of empowerment, enabling better control of our emotional lives, is valuable for everyone."

To learn more, please visit peterla mbrou.com.

Dr. Lipton said that to break free of the programming, you have to first recognize that your subconscious mind exists. You must accept that the manifestation of limitations or disease is because of what's happening in the field of invisible subconscious programs. (Although he also recognizes that about 3 to 5 percent of disease is due to "birth defects"—alteration of the genetic code that occurred before birth.)

That's the hard part, because, of course, you say to yourself, "I wouldn't create this!" Anyone who has been through diseases such as cancer bristles at this idea, because we absolutely would *not* create the situation consciously. Dr. Lipton, however, urges us to consider that the subconscious mind has been running programs that most likely brought the cancer on. He says that before we can begin the work of really healing, first we must let go of guilt and self-blame—after all, we were downloaded with limiting behavioral programs in our childhood without our conscious awareness.

"You can rewire yourself," he said. "If a disease such as cancer has progressed to an advanced stage, then you might do a round or two of chemo, but at the same time you need to be reprogramming your mind and recognizing your involvement in the disease. You must recognize that you are a participant in the unfolding of your life. Then you can go into your subconscious program and find out where the problems are."

Dr. Lipton's research suggests that the subconscious mind is built on habituation. It learns from patterns and repetition of patterns. By accessing that invisible field, you can rewrite those habits. The million-dollar question is, how?

According to Dr. Lipton, we can do this in many ways. "Through processes such as hypnosis, subliminal tapes, the religious use of affirmations, Buddhist mindfulness, or a series of reprogramming modalities collectively referred to as energy psychology, such as PSYCH-K, Emotional Self-Management (ESM), Eye Movement Desensitization and Reprocessing (EMDR), and Emotional Freedom Techniques (EFT), among many other new techniques, we can rewrite those destructive programs that occupy our subconscious field."

The core of Dr. Lipton's premise is that by rewiring the subconscious thoughts that negatively impact our cells, we have a far greater chance of healing. The absence of doing this kind of work could also explain why cancer recurs, even after hard-core treatment and years of remission.

Science, said Dr. Lipton, is onboard with the platform of epigenetics, even though most of modern medicine disregards it. Given the profound implications of his research, and the evidence he's witnessed that proves its merit, it seems unbelievable that the medical world rejects it. But that's the point; medical professionals don't want to believe it.

"The amount of money you have invested in a belief system ('Doctors have the authority; I am ruled by my genes; drugs are the only cure') determines how willing you are to change it. The financial investment we have in medicine—and especially pharmaceutical drugs—is far too high for those factions to make a change. They don't want change, no matter how much good it could do.

"Medical institutions are operating on fear. The funding and regulatory elements know that within each of us is the power to heal. For example, it is a proven fact that one-third of all healings are due to the placebo effect, which is controlled by the mind, but medical-related corporations based on making a profit don't want us to know this. It's interesting that more than 85 percent of doctors don't even belong to the policy-making professional union called the American Medical Association. That means that the decisions made by 10 percent of the US medical community control the outcome of the entire medical profession. They determine standard practices, but they're controlled by investors. And the FDA is heavily invested in the pharmaceutical business."[1]

It's curious to contemplate if an entire industry can possess a subconscious mind. Ideally, people go into medicine because they want to help other people. Yet, the very system in which they work can block those good intentions, since they can only pull from a very limited pool of (FDA-approved)

---

[1] The AMA claims membership of approximately 30 percent of people who practice medicine.

resources, when in fact there exists a wide range of viable alternatives. If there is a sabotaging belief in the subconscious mind of the drug industry, I wonder what it would be, and how it could be exhumed.

Political dynamics are nothing new in the world of medicine, as Dr. Lipton described: "Back in 1925, physicists discovered that everything in the universe is based on energy—not matter. Everything physicists thought they knew had to be revised. In other words, consciousness is primary in creating the world. They went from believing in the *machine* itself to what *runs* the machine, but they couldn't yet take it into the world; it was too radical an idea for the public to accept. Therefore, they arbitrarily agreed to restrict the principles of quantum physics to the realm of atoms and not bring it into the realm of people, societies, or communities."

Given the politics of medicine, I asked Dr. Lipton where science and spirituality actually intersect. "Quantum physics," he replied with confidence. "The definition of spirit is 'an invisible moving force that influences life or matter.' Einstein said, 'The Field is the sole governing agency of the particle.' According to physicists, the Field is defined as exactly the same thing: 'an invisible moving force that influences life or matter.' As it turns out, the Field and spirit are the same. The observer creates reality."

After observing his own reality and admitting to difficulties in his personal life, Dr. Lipton pursued rewiring his own subconscious programs. Although he spoke as a scientist, his passion flowed from personal experience. "I was living a life of folly. I went in and out of trusting this stuff—all of which I've now come to know as true. Being a teacher, I had to learn it, but I had grave doubts. I went through some very tough times at first. Then, when I needed something, and I asked God (the Field) to give it to me, something would come forth. I'd say, 'Show me something,' and the universe would show me. Finally, I had to own it. Now, I don't know what the future will bring, but I know that folly doesn't work. Now I live in a wonderful reality.

"There's a force moving within us, a biological imperative to survive and to avoid death. It's built in. Right now, there's the question of our own extinction, and none of us want to die."

What is it in the subconscious mind of the individual—or the collective whole—that takes us to the brink of destruction? Only through entering the world of the subconscious mind's programming will we find out. "I was living in a self-imposed world that resembled purgatory," Dr. Lipton recalled in a quiet voice. "I thought, 'What the hell is wrong with this world?' Now I'm walking in heaven. I've recognized who I really am and have rewritten the limiting programs that disempowered me."

The new science of epigenetics promises that every person on the planet has the opportunity to become who they really are, complete with unimaginable power and the ability to operate from, and go for, the highest possibilities, including healing our bodies and our culture and living in peace.

***

Dr. Bruce Lipton received the 2009 Goi Peace Award "in recognition of his pioneering work in the field of New Biology, and his outstanding contribution toward the realization of a peaceful and harmonious world for all life on earth."

To learn more about Dr. Lipton, go to brucelipton.com. See the appendix for a full listing of Dr. Lipton's books and CDs. To learn more about the Goi Peace Award, see goipeace.or.jp.

The thing that is really hard, and really amazing, is giving up on being perfect and beginning the work of becoming yourself.

ANNA QUINDLEN

CHAPTER 6

Belief

Ask, and it will be given you; Seek, and you will find; Knock, and it will be opened to you.
MATTHEW 7:7

It's ironic that a chapter about belief may be hard for people to believe. Believing is a tricky business. Here's what I believe.

Beliefs are the gateway to opportunity or obstacle, freedom or bondage. Belief systems are unconscious prayers. Essentially, whatever we believe is an unwitting request to a very generous God who wants to give us whatever we ask for. Our thoughts create the tone, or vibration, that dwells within our bodies. God responds to that vibration.

In the most simplistic of terms, if we see the world as a place full of nasty people who do malicious things, we maintain a tone that attracts people who are unkind and deceitful, therefore creating our reality just as we believe it is. Likewise, if we perceive the world as safe, loving, and friendly, peopled by souls that are inherently good, then we maintain a tone that projects this, and the Divine Source will cast our world with kind and compassionate people who act with love in their hearts just as we do. And so it is.

It doesn't matter what we believe: God graciously presents us with people and circumstances that reflect the story of whatever we believe. If you don't believe this, chances are you will not experience the elegance, simplicity, or grace of it. Rather, you will probably see yourself as a victim of people and circumstances, with no power to change what goes on in your life. That is your belief, and so it will be.

Free will equals the freedom to believe whatever we want. Those beliefs translate into a cosmic platform that God wants to accommodate. It all goes back to those old sayings "You get what you give" or "What goes around comes around."

This is relevant for everyone, but especially when you want to heal from cancer. As mentioned earlier, everyone's heard of the placebo effect. People are given a sugar pill to cure some dreaded disease, and somehow it cures the dreaded disease. The sugar pill was a tool that the belief system latched onto, and healing occurred.

The opposite of that is the nocebo effect. As Dr. Bruce Lipton said, the nocebo effect is when someone tells us something bad is going to happen, such as "You're going to die"; your belief system attaches to the idea that "I'm going to die"; and then all kinds of things go about making it so.

"Reality is in the mind of the believer," I once heard myself say, as I inched through the clanking, clinical tunnel of an MRI machine. By then, I had come to know that the brawn behind our beliefs determines the quality and circumstances of our lives. I was working hard on changing mine. I was, after all, desperately trying to contradict the nocebo effect that had started to work on me. Suddenly, my job was to release all the beliefs that I had inherited from the world about cancer, starting with, "I don't have to die from this," then moving to the fact that I could find my way to full and complete healing.

Thoughts and beliefs are not made of stone, which means they should be easy to change, right? Well, of course, it all depends on what you believe, but here's what I experienced: it's easy to say, "I can heal cancer with natural remedies; I can do it by sending my cells loving energy, by using visualization, and by feeding them good, nutritious foods." That's easy to say, but to actually *believe* it to the core of your soul is quite another task. In fact, truly believing it without doubt or hesitation can feel like pulling a train out of quicksand.

That's because along with every idea is a *train of thought* attached to or associated with a bigger thought. When I decided that I could heal my cancer, a boxcar of thoughts appeared and shouted, "That's such bull! You can't do that. You can use only chemo and radiation, which, by the way, will put you through hell and probably won't work. Plus, cells are impacted by genes, not by the food you eat or the thoughts you think. All this stuff about your emotional well-being impacting your cells is just a bunch of New Age hooey. Get a life."

This boxcar of thoughts then required that I release each thought in order to create a different, more generative belief system that would feed into my goal of healing.

Then came the next boxcar. It was loaded with: "But what if I can't do it? What if it's true, but I just don't ever figure out how to do it? What if it only works for some people and not others? Wait, it's supposed to work for everyone, so why not me? Do I have a death wish? Do I have what it takes? I probably don't have what it takes." And so on.

Finding a way to believe in things you have not believed in before—especially when you think your life might be at stake—demands the most steadfast mental discipline you will ever know. It's a constant dance in the head, one that shimmies and twists in the most confounding manner.

You can think you're doing great, dwelling in the peace and trust of your newfound conviction, when all of a sudden, BAM! Another boxcar of fearful, mistrusting thoughts derails you: "You're in denial, you know. Anyone with any sense knows that cancer isn't controllable this way. Everyone knows that it's a disease on its own destructive path with no mercy, even for well-meaning people like you."

Needless to say, the work continues. Even now, years later, I recognize thoughts rooted deep within that I need to bring to light and set free so I can make way for all the goodness I desire for myself. It's hard to believe that our thoughts and beliefs have so much power; I continue to have moments, even days, of doubt.

However, as I look deeply at my own life, as I accept responsibility for creating both what we call good stuff and what we call bad, I can't help but see something huge. It's bigger than the train of thoughts. It's bigger than what our society, our sciences, or many of our churches recognize. It's tucked deeply within each of us. *It is our own unique power.* It is the source of our creative genius, and it is from the

Source of all creation. It is our direct connection to God. It is in this place that our thoughts and beliefs get circulated, and come back to us as the realities we live out.

When we realize this, we pay much closer attention to the thoughts and feelings we entertain. We respect that the quality and nature of the vibration within will come back to give us either what we want or what we fear and resist the most.

Strong belief systems penetrate every corner of the medical world. Indeed, the most glowing difference between the doctors I have spoken with, those who oversee alternative treatments, and those who administer allopathic protocols, is in what they believe.

There is practical evidence that all types of treatments can work, but most mainstream medical doctors don't believe in alternatives. They believe only in what they have to offer. After a point, if their own therapies fail, they believe there is nothing more to do. They don't believe in anything else; therefore, they see death.

Alternative practitioners believe in their therapies, and they have seen them work. Alternative doctors believe there is much to be done, and in most cases, there is hope. They believe it; therefore, they see it.

What happens to us is evidence of what we believe in. This truth sheds light on the fact that it's not just our conscious thoughts that send messages to the universe; it's largely our subconscious thoughts as well. This is why we can think positively until we're blue in the face, and still end up with circumstances that we don't want. This is why it's so important to pay attention to the resolution of whatever subconscious beliefs may be intruding on what we think we want. This is why it's important to believe in the ability to penetrate the complexities of our minds.

As you embark on your healing, believe in your path fully. No matter what treatment you choose, invest time, energy, meditation, and as many waking hours as possible in believing that they will work. Pray that they will. Pray daily that you believe they will.

A person who doubts himself is like a man who would enlist in the ranks of his enemies and bear arms against himself.
ALEXANDRE DUMAS

ISSA'S STORY

You may never know what results come from your action. But if you do nothing, there will be no result.
MAHATMA GANDHI

Issa likes it when things can be explained scientifically. As a college professor, he's comfortable with academia and the rules of cause and effect. That's also why he followed his doctor's advice to treat his metastatic prostate cancer in the manner that medical science deemed most promising.

"The cancer was in 90 percent of my prostate," Issa recalled, "and also in parts of my sacrum. Plus, my abdominal lymph nodes looked suspicious, as did spots in my kidney and liver. They told me I had two to three years to live, and they immediately put me on conventional therapy. Because the cancer had metastasized, it didn't make sense to do chemo, radiation, or surgery. Instead, I was put on a double hormonal blockade. They administered a subcutaneous injection of a hormone blocker, Zoladex, which lasted three months, and in addition prescribed Casodex. The hormone blocker shut down the entire male hormone system with the purpose of slowing down the spread of the cancer. Even so, they told me that eventually the cancer would adapt and outmaneuver the hormone ablation therapy. At that point, they'd try throwing chemo and radiation at it."

And that would be it.

Meanwhile, Issa's wife, who knew something about the importance of diet, had been researching other available possibilities for her husband. That's when she came across the Gerson Therapy (see page 186). She compared it to other diet-based treatments and decided that it was both scientifically and biologically sound.

"Within a month, we were practicing the Gerson Therapy," Issa reported. "After a year of being on the diet, I asked my urologist to do an MRI. This was in September 2003, exactly one year to the date of my diagnosis. He resisted because he figured the cancer would still be there, given that the hormone treatment doesn't cure the cancer. The doctor who finally agreed to the scan was one of the best in the field and used state-of-the-art MRI technology. There wasn't one speck of cancer anywhere—not in the prostate, nor anywhere else. They were stunned."

After a year on the Gerson Therapy, Issa was cancer free, but he continued with the hormonal therapy for another year and a half. "I was told by the Gerson people that the blockers would interfere with the Gerson Therapy, but I did it anyway. I was too cautious. At the same time, I also committed 100 percent to the diet for nearly three years. After my third cancer-free MRI in May 2005, I finally got off the hormonal blocks."

The Gerson Therapy is intense and rigorous, but Issa's commitment was unyielding. He monitored his blood quarterly and reached PSA levels of 0.6 and 0.8 (normal is anything below 4.0).

He juiced regularly and did the required number of coffee enemas.

Given the severe restrictions of the diet, I asked Issa how he was able to follow it so faithfully. "I asked for a semester off from teaching, and the school held the position for me. My wife and I had established a business in our home so that I could do the therapy at home. We devoted all of our time to the therapy. We were fortunate because we had both the time and the financial means to do it. But really, whether you're in that kind of position or not, it can be done. We were organized and disciplined. We didn't care about a social life. This was about life or death. Within two months, we knew it was working. It was amazing, really amazing. The cancer was cured as though it had never been there."

Issa admitted that it took some self-awareness for him to commit to the program, but when he understood the scientific logic of the therapy, he was able to adopt a strong and certain conviction. As Issa explained it, the science behind the Gerson Therapy works like this: the diet essentially strengthens the immune, hormone, and enzyme systems. It restores functions to the organs by flooding the body with rapidly metabolizing nutrients. With such an intense intake of nutrients, along with constant detoxification, the body restores the immune system to its peak level, and the immune system then attacks and eliminates the cancer.

Issa said, "The therapy's components comprise a coherent, interdependent, unitary system, and are based on solid scientific logic. These components, such as the salt-to-potassium ratio, have been independently, scientifically analyzed. The juices provide massive intakes of macro and micronutrients, which, along with the initial strictly vegetarian diet, provide oxidative enzymes that enhance the oxygen supply to the cells. Then you manage the potassium-to-salt ratio to essentially make sure you have virtually no salt. You have high levels of potassium and low levels of sodium, which expel cancer from the cells. You also have to keep your thyroid-hormone function at optimum levels. The management and relationship of these things is massively important."

The therapy also limits fats and animal proteins because these turn on the cancer receptors, and fat comes largely from animal products. The Gerson Therapy (and most other cancer-fighting diets) totally omits fats and animal proteins, certainly in the early stages of the therapy. Finally, the therapy uses large intakes of metabolic enzymes, in addition to niacin, and requires B12/crude liver injections, important in restoring tissues and new red blood corpuscles. There is also no use of processed foods, oils, or sugars.

"You put all these things together, and you have an incredibly effective scientific system. I looked through all the literature of those who call it ineffective, and I decided that there's just a lot of ignorance out there. If scientists call this bogus, then they're not being scientific; they're not showing scientific curiosity and are ignoring the thousands of people who've been cured from cancer and other degenerative diseases. They should absolutely subject this regimen to scientific testing and studies."

At the time he was engaged in and committed to his healing, Issa's mother and two nieces died of cancer. "The people I know that did conventional therapy have died. The ones who have committed to this program invariably see improvement and a retreat of the cancer. But everyone has to do their own thing. I know that time and money come into play, but if you really want to, you can organize this treatment as the core of your life and get rid of your cancer. I can't imagine why people wouldn't want to do this to save their lives."

Given Issa's preference for scientific data, I was curious about his thoughts on why people get cancer. "From the research I did," he said, "it's all pretty much outlined in *The China Study* by Dr. T. Colin Campbell. It's our meat-eating diet and our lifestyle, along with environmental factors such as pollution."

Scientific data illustrates how diet plays into prostate cancer. Only about 10 percent of men who live (and eat) in Mediterranean and Asian countries get prostate cancer. When those same healthy men move to the United States and adopt the standard American diet, their incidence of cancer increases overwhelmingly.

What Is Food?

"Your body needs real food." Even though it sounds like a no-brainer, that's the advice of Nancy Deville, author of *Death by Supermarket.* That said, Deville is the first to admit that reforming from a diet of fake food to a diet of real food means paying attention and taking action. Clean out your kitchen of all factory food products, and stock it with real food. Mute TV food commercials, question what your doctor recommends, and rebel against some well-established "truths."

"Our bodies need real food," she told me, "because we're made up of the components in food. Since our bodies are constantly breaking down and building back up, it makes sense that we need to provide the building materials for these processes. But we've become convinced by the food industry, government, and the medical community that eating artificial food is OK, even healthy.

"Food 'products' are not real food. Contrary to what we're led to believe, many things we ingest aren't safe, including fake butter, soy products, and tap water. Fake dairy creamer is so bizarre that it makes me wonder how in the world it could end up, say, on a hospital food tray. Commercial milk is toxic and one of the causes of the rise in cancers. On the other hand, raw milk from cows that eat grass is a perfect food. The difference is very important to understand. These days, we have to be like our ancient ancestors and learn how to avoid poisons and forage for healthy sustenance."

It may sound extreme, but Deville isn't shooting blanks. Her book documents scientific evidence to back up her claims. Hers and other books, such as *The Whole Soy Story: The Dark Side of America's Favorite Health*

Food by Kaayla T. Daniel; *The Raw Truth About Milk* by William Campbell Douglass II; and *Nutrition and Physical Degeneration* by Andrew Weston, tell a different story than the ones we're used to hearing.

Even though you're responsible for what you put in your mouth, Deville maintains that people with cancer should not blame themselves for getting sick. "We're getting more cancer because our environment is inundated with carcinogens, but you can do things to eliminate some of what fuels the cancer. Don't drink diet sodas or ingest anything 'diet.' If you look at the label of a food product and there is gobbledygook that requires a biochemical degree to understand, it makes sense that this is not food; it's something cooked up in a laboratory with chemicals that are bad for human beings. I'm talking about things Americans love, like microwavable junk, cold cereal (even the health-food kind), and chemically processed polyunsaturated omega-6 fats, among others."

Deville encourages people to pay attention to the symptoms we've come to think are normal. "People think they can put whatever they want into their bodies, and it will process everything and come out the other end. It doesn't work that way. If you have gastrointestinal problems, it's your body telling you, 'I don't like what you're putting in me!' If you're gaining weight, you have dark circles under your eyes, your hair is thinning, your nails are brittle, you're constipated, you have constant headaches, and you are fatigued, look at your diet. Does it start in the morning with sugar? Is that followed by some dead, low-fat crud like a diet TV dinner? If so, pretty soon your body begins to break down, and you see the evidence of the breakdown in the mirror."

The food industry fattens us up, Deville said, then the drug and diet industries step in to profit from the obesity and disease caused by a fake food diet. "The diet industry would absolutely hate it if Americans got healthy, because then they would stop dieting. If you want to stay unhealthy, keep dieting. If you want to lose weight, stop dieting and start eating a regular diet of only real food. It's a very simple formula. As long as we continue to diet and eat fake food, we stay dependent on over-the-counter drugs. We take something in the morning for one symptom, then another in the afternoon for another symptom, then at night we pop something else. Pretty soon, we're taking six or seven drugs every day. Eating fake food, dieting, and taking drug cocktails is a recipe for metabolic disaster, and I'm talking fat, disease, and depression."

Deville's advice is to *get educated.*

"Read, read, read. If you have cancer, read Dr. Russell Blaylock's book, *Natural Strategies for Cancer Patients.* Sign up for his newsletter and learn how to give your body what it needs to fight cancer. Explore the literature that is out there on natural health. It's all over the place, and now there is no excuse for anyone to remain in the dark.

"To make it very simple, just think in terms of what people ate historically—foods that were picked, gathered, milked, hunted, or fished. We need to go back to primitive thinking when it comes to food. When you look for food in the grocery store, ask yourself, 'What has been done to this food?' If it's in an unnatural state, don't eat it.

"Don't be hysterical about it, though," said Deville. "You can't always eat perfectly, because our environment prevents it. When we're scared and worried, we tend to go off the deep end with radical diet approaches. Heal your body cell by cell with a consistent diet of real food.

"If some poison sneaks in, don't beat yourself up. Just have something real the next meal."

To learn more about Nancy Deville and her books, go to nancydeville.com. For additional book recommendations on diet and cancer, see the appendix.

I then asked Issa about the mind-body connection, and if he believes it may have helped to cure his own cancer. He said, "That's incidental to the therapy. The Gerson Therapy is the foundation. There is no question that attitude affects our proneness to or avoidance of disease. A negative attitude can suppress the immune system, and that can be shown chemically. I think of the mind-body connection as a complement to the Gerson Therapy. Of course, it's good to meditate and access your spiritual life. That calms you down and helps you, if you believe it can get rid of the disease."

Even though Issa's perception of healing is clearly rooted in the physical, he did acknowledge that his mindset contributed to why he got the disease. "There was probably a genetic tendency in my case, but one of my flaws was carrying the world on my shoulders. I had a tendency toward melancholy and depression. I do think this led to the cancer. Yes, intuitively I know that my attitude led to this cancer."

These days, years after his doctors gave him little hope, Issa's outlook is brighter because of his experience with cancer and what was required to heal. "I have a different attitude about life and its many facets. It changed me dramatically, but over time we tend to go back to old habits. I try to remind myself and resurrect the self-awareness that came out of this experience. Something spectacular happened. I was given a second chance. And even though I'm not the type of person who goes through life happy, content, and elated, things have improved."

The Gerson Therapy, according to Issa, has the logical and scientific platform that's necessary to heal. He cautions people that they don't have to spend lots of money on alternative care; for instance, he never actually visited the Gerson Institute. With the help of his wife, he learned and did the therapy on his own. He bought the books that guided him through the Gerson Therapy, bought the equipment necessary to carry it out, and committed fully to it. "You cannot hover between one therapy and another," he said. "Not if you want to do a serious alternative."

Issa has been married for twenty-seven years and reports that all of the sexual abilities that were temporarily destroyed during his conventional treatment have returned. To some men with prostate cancer, this may be among the best reasons to consider the Gerson approach to healing.

Many things which cannot be overcome when they are together yield themselves up when taken little by little.
PLUTARCH

CHARLOTTE GERSON

The Gerson Institute

To change one's life: 1. Start immediately. 2. Do it flamboyantly. 3. No exceptions.
WILLIAM JAMES

Charlotte Gerson has minced truckloads of garlic in her eighty-eight years of life, but I'd venture to say she's rarely minced her words. Her opinions are strong, and her advice is passionate. That's because since she was a young girl growing up in Germany, she both experienced and witnessed what would be called "miraculous healings" of people with an array of what are considered fatal illnesses.

"In this toxic world, you're going to get toxic," she told me in a heavy German accent that emphasized her point. "If you are not healthy, you will die."

Charlotte's primary defense against that doomed fate is food. Not just any food, though. It's got to be fresh, organic fruits and vegetables—lots of them—and for those who are sick, those foods must be prepared in ways that offer the body the most promise for regaining homeostasis.

To understand the Gerson Therapy and why Charlotte's convictions run so deep, you first have to go back not just to her childhood, but to her father's childhood as well. In 1888, when German-born Max Gerson was seven years old, he was playing in his grandmother's garden. She was experimenting with fertilizers. On one side of the garden, she tilled in her organic fertilizer, while on the other side she applied a newly developed artificial fertilizer. Max noticed (and never forgot) that the worms in the soil of the artificial fertilizer migrated to the soil with the organic matter. It meant nothing to him at the time, but decades later it would symbolize a beautifully simple premise: nature prefers and thrives in unadulterated environments.

Max became a doctor and, like most people trained in the medical field, knew nothing about nutrition. So at age twenty-five, when he experienced incapacitating migraine headaches, it didn't occur to him to change his diet. His doctor assured him that he would outgrow the headaches by the time he reached his midfifties. For this young, ambitious doctor, waiting twenty-five years was out of the question.

In a determined search to find the cure, he learned of a woman who had cured her migraines by changing her diet. Dr. Gerson decided to drink only milk—nothing more—and see if that helped. On the contrary, it worsened the condition. He then began researching the diets of our ancestors and soon opted to eat a diet solely of apples. The migraines vanished. Over time, he introduced more foods into his system and eventually created what he called his "migraine diet." It consisted of organic fruits and vegetables, as well as bountiful amounts of their juices.

After his own cure, Dr. Gerson suggested the diet to a patient who also suffered from migraines. Upon following his orders, one woman was delighted to report that not only were her migraines gone, so was the tuberculosis (TB) she had suffered on parts of her skin. Dr. Gerson was shocked because he had thought that TB was incurable.

After conferring with Professor Ferdinand Sauerbruch, a famous TB specialist, Sauerbruch offered to test this dietary approach on 450 seriously ill skin-TB patients. Of those tested, 446 recovered. Subsequently, Dr. Gerson prescribed the diet to other patients suffering from TB, among them the wife of Nobel Prize winner Dr. Albert Schweitzer, who suffered from lung TB.

Charlotte also became the benefactor of her father's knowledge, because she was also cured of TB.

Dr. Gerson was beginning to recognize that when the body's immune system is fully nurtured, it doesn't only heal a single condition—it heals them all. But his rigorous scientific mind still wasn't satisfied. His new approach to testing the diet was to accept only patients who were told by at least three different doctors that they were incurable. The patients who came to him experienced a wide range of ailments, including secondary problems such as allergies, high blood pressure, asthma, and more. After undergoing Dr. Gerson's therapy, however, all of their problems ceased to exist, and his pod of "incurable" patients walked back into their lives free of physical drama.

This was the point at which Dr. Gerson understood the magnificence of the human body. Without question, he knew that the body has healing powers within, when and if it is given proper nutrients. This was also the point at which Dr. Gerson started to veer away from the traditions and thinking of mainstream medicine.

"He was attacked from every which way," recalled Charlotte. "He threatened the very foundation of financial solvency in the medical world. When the war came, he had plenty of reasons to relocate, so with the help of someone in New York whom he had cured, we moved to the United States." Dr. Gerson was classically educated and knew Latin and Greek, but not English. Upon arriving here, he embarked upon learning the language so that he could pass the tests that would earn him a medical license.

While still in France and before arriving in the U.S., Dr. Gerson met a doctor who ran a camp for children with bone cancer. The diet was introduced to the children, and they began to heal. This wasn't exactly what the attending physician was after. In confidence, he asked Dr. Gerson, "If we heal all of these children, what will become of us?"

The therapy was stopped.

"What can you say about that?" Charlotte asked, which brings us back to her vigor as she spoke about the cancer industry. "It didn't take long for the FDA and AMA to take notice of my father. They didn't like what they saw, and they pegged him as a fraud and a quack. You see, when you use organic fruits and vegetables to heal cancer, you make no money from it. You can't patent food, so they use chemo instead, which admittedly causes cancer."

Charlotte said that even doctors who administer chemo often don't use it. She cited a survey given to oncologists, in which they were asked if they would use chemo on themselves or a loved one in the case of cancer. Sixty-four percent of the doctors said no. "What does that tell you?" Charlotte went on. "It's a big business.

"Dr. Ralph Moss, who used to work at Sloan Kettering, states in his book, *The Cancer Industry,* that the cancer industry made $100 billion per year in the US alone.[1] That was in 1989. I'm not being cynical; it's simply mathematics. It's a fact. These days, the cancer industry is worth far more than that."

I asked Charlotte why more doctors don't step up and speak out about the poor success rate of mainstream treatment and the promise of the Gerson Therapy. "We've healed doctors and their family members, but they ask us not to use their names. Medical students start their career about $100,000 in debt. If they don't do what they're told, they can lose their license. The California Health Department says that any doctor who uses anything other than chemo, radiation, and surgery in the diagnosis or treatment of cancer could be convicted of a felony, lose their license, pay a $10,000 fine, or even go to jail. Do you think any doctor would go outside the system? No. They are financial slaves."

That said, Charlotte didn't claim that the Gerson Therapy works for everyone. "When the immune system is fully operational, it doesn't heal selectively. When you restore the enzymes, minerals, and other nutrients, you heal everything. That means when you heal the cancer, you also heal the diabetes. When you truly heal, the whole body heals. Our patients come to us with many diseases and carry on to fully restore the body's defenses and defeat all their diseases. This is a huge threat to the multibillion-dollar pharmaceutical industry."

Charlotte's passion surfaced without reserve when she talked about the business behind the cancer industry. "Pharmacies are retail outlets. Big Pharma controls the FDA and other government organizations. You know how much it costs to run for any political office? Millions. Who do you think pays for that? Pharmaceutical companies are among the richest in the world. They have trillions of dollars. Change will never come from above because they're happy with their money and power."

Given that food is the medicine behind the Gerson Therapy, I asked how the government controls our food. She laughed. "The FDA has approved about ten thousand food additives they say are safe. How come if you eat those foods, you get sick, but if you eat only fresh organic foods, you can cure the incurable?"

She also says the alarming rise of cancer among children is a result of poor diet, MSG (monosodium glutamate), and the use of microwaves, which she says destroy nutrients. "Kids are the new market for doctors," she adds.

The FDA and AMA may control the business that's behind medicine; the good news, however, is that each one of us controls what we put in our mouths. According to Charlotte, that's a choice we all must make, yet it's not necessarily easy to make the wisest choice. "I prepare all of my own food," she said. "I drive eighteen miles to a store that sells organic foods. I never eat in restaurants. In this toxic world, I do everything I can so that at least the food I eat is clean. I'm eighty-eight years old, and I take no drugs, no hormones. And I have no arthritis, no high blood pressure, nothing. I'm fine. There isn't a single number in my blood count or urinalysis that's out of range."

That may be why her mind is so sharp. Indeed, Charlotte claimed that *negative thinking is due to undernourished brain cells.* At the same time, she admitted that positive thoughts can contribute to healing. "Prayer and meditation make a difference, but I can't tell you how much. The mind is a powerful instrument. By all means, use it."

Still, Charlotte believes the toxins in our world are largely responsible for disease. "Half of all cancers are caused by environmental toxicity. The other half are caused by deficiency. To get well, you must first detoxify your body so that your organs are restored, then eat very selectively with living nutrients. The treatment for an advanced cancer patient, which requires fresh juice every hour and proper preparation of fresh, organic foods, is very work intensive. The patient needs help for the long hours of work."

This may sound impractical, but if your prognosis is grim and you have time and the necessary help, the Gerson Therapy offers a regiment of hope and freedom from disease.

The Particulars

Where: The Gerson Clinic, Baja Nutri Care, is located in the beach area of Tijuana, Mexico (Playas de Tijuana).

Administrative offices are located in San Diego.

Who: Licensed physicians with long-term Gerson experience are on hand. A doctor and nurse are on the premises twenty-four hours a day, every day.

What to expect: They'll ask for your latest medical records to make sure your situation is appropriate for their protocol. (People who have undergone an organ transplant or are on kidney dialysis are ineligible.)

Blood tests, X-rays, and urinalysis tests are conducted at US licensed laboratories. The clinic avoids tests that require dyes or the injection of chemicals. It conducts tests to make sure your kidneys and liver enzymes are functioning.

Patients consume 10 to 13 fresh, organic juices daily. Each patient is taught how to prepare the juices and food. Patients attend lectures, watch food demonstrations, and leave with an understanding of what they need to do.

To detoxify, patients take 3 to 5 coffee enemas daily.

Noticeable changes can occur in 24 to 36 hours.

The menu is strictly controlled. The foods are both cooked and raw, although specific foods are prohibited, including sugar, salt, soybeans and their derivatives, animal protein, all oils except flaxseed oil, and especially all prepared and processed foods.

Once people go home, they continue the protocol. Patients can return anytime they want. Many return to encourage new patients by showing how they are in good condition after the treatment.

Typical routine: The strict routine is thoroughly described in Charlotte Gerson's most recent book, *Healing the Gerson Way,* available from Totality Books (831-625-3565) and the Gerson Institute.

Since rest is an important part of healing, exercise is strictly limited, especially for the seriously ill patients. Rest and early sleep are important; however, entertainment is highly valuable as well, especially anything humorous and light in nature.

Where to stay: Participants stay on site at the clinic, twenty-four hours a day for three weeks. Each of the ten rooms has two beds, one for the patient and one for a companion. Each room has a private bathroom. Companions are required, and the companion's room and board are included in the cost. It is essential for patients to bring a person who will learn the therapy with them, witness the positive results in other patients, and help the patients when they get home.

Cost: $5,500 per week. Charge includes all meals and juices, Gerson medications, doctor and nurse visits, lectures, food- and juice-preparation instruction, books, weekly blood and urinalysis tests, and companion's room and board.

Who goes: Patients come from all over the world. It is important that either the patients or their companions speak English or Spanish, so they can communicate with the doctors and nurses. By far, the largest majority of patients arriving at the Gerson Clinic are in "terminal condition." Those who have not yet been treated by chemo and radiation respond more easily to the Gerson Therapy. There are also many patients with heart disease, diabetes, rheumatoid arthritis, colitis, fibromyalgia, and many other conditions that respond positively to the Gerson Therapy. The therapy generally does not work for people affected by Parkinson's, Huntington's chorea, and ALS (amystrophic lateral sclerosis, or Lou Gehrig's Disease).

Words of wisdom: "It's such a joy to go to our hospital," Charlotte said, with rare levity in her voice. "We get almost exclusively terminally ill patients who have had the cancer come back after chemo and radiation. When they come to us, they can hardly eat, they're nauseated, and it's hard. After one week, however, they are piling their plates high with fresh food and laughing and joking. That's the picture of healing.

"Dr. Schweitzer himself was cured of type 2 diabetes after eating the Gerson diet. When my father died decades later, Dr. Schweitzer said, 'I see in him one of the most eminent geniuses in the history of medicine. Many of his basic ideas have been adopted without having his name connected with them. Yet he has achieved more than seemed possible under adverse conditions. He leaves a legacy which commands attention and which will assure him his due place. Those whom he has cured will now attest to the truth of his ideas.'"

Contact Information:

The Gerson Institute/Cancer Curing
 Society
1572 Second Avenue
San Diego, CA 92101
619-685-5353/888-443-7766 (US only)
800-838-2256 (US and Canada)
Fax: 619-685-5363
gerson.org

The Noah rule: predicting rain doesn't count; building arks does.
WARREN BUFFETT

CHAPTER 7

Gratitude

One day in retrospect the years of struggle will strike you as the most beautiful.
SIGMUND FREUD

I used to be so limber that during yoga classes I would surprise even myself. Of course, I had nothing over the yoga teachers, but for a regular middle-aged chick, I did pretty darn well.

I recently began practicing yoga again, more than two years after the surgery that forever altered my body. Things are different now. Radiation has ravaged my hips; they're stiff and inflexible, and they cramp easily. I can open only them so far before a biting pain takes over. I am unable to do some of the most basic poses that were once as easy as waving hello. My body is not what it used to be. It is truly limited.

In my yoga class today, while everyone else twisted one leg over the other, giving the opposing hip a good stretch—such a simple posture—I winced in pain until the teacher whispered, "Don't do it. It's too much." Then I started to cry, and I couldn't stop.

There are many losses in life, and after a cancer diagnosis—and some of the treatments—there can be so many so fast. It was apparent years ago, right after my course of radiation, that my hips were locked up with scar tissue. But not until the yoga class did it hit me in the way that losing your identity and then having to redefine yourself hits you.

At the end of the class, as we lay prone, relaxing our bodies, the tears kept coming. This time I was surprised not at how limber I was, but at how deeply this had affected me. I was grieving.

But then I surrendered to the greatest lesson I have learned since all this came down: to be grateful.

"I used to be physically limber and emotionally stiff," I heard my inner self say. "Now I'm physically locked up, but emotionally limber." I felt some measure of relief.

Then I asked myself who or what I was mad at for this condition. The cancer? No. Dr. R., my radiologist? Kind of. I wanted to blame him—anyone—for this limitation.

"But no," I thought, "he's doing what he thinks is best to help people. The radiation? Yes, I'm mad at the radiation. OK, then. More forgiveness work on the way."

In truth, I'm the one that I have to forgive for agreeing to do the procedure that brought all this about. And I will, because I was doing what I thought was best to help myself.

Gratitude, I've learned, can fish us out of the deepest reservoir of despair. I didn't know that before. Instead, I lived wrapped tightly under the sharp scrutiny of a discerning eye. My habit was to look for what needed to be improved, beautified, discarded, altered, or changed in any number of ways to make it, or my perception of it, better. I was unaware that by living that way, I was living out of lack, which is a stepchild of fear. Nothing was ever quite good enough because I rarely took notice of what was very good indeed. Rather, I gave my attention elsewhere, feeling completely justified because after my makeover, things would surly improve. Sometimes they did. And if I were paying attention to something I couldn't "fix," such as the crime rate or inept government, I would talk for hours on end with Eddie or my friends about the horrible injustices that surrounded us.

Even though I was an upbeat person, I had the perpetual glass-half-empty syndrome, which I hadn't known about myself until my world was turned upside down, and I suddenly saw the glass as half full—well, maybe even completely full. Or better yet, brimming over.

The shift took place when I understood that I might fall into the great abyss. Indeed, my toes were curled over the precipice of this life, and my balance was tenuous. This is a vantage point that rocks the hell out of you. When you think it's all about to disappear, when you think you're about to lose it all, lose your very breath and heartbeat, suddenly, perhaps for the first time, you see everything you could lose—which is everything you have, which is so very, very much.

As I continue to heal (because the layers of the onion will always present us with something more!), I have come to know that being grateful or appreciative and paying attention to the bounty of blessings before us is, along with forgiveness, perhaps the greatest key to inner peace and freedom.

Each loss we experience steals our full attention. These losses often beckon anger or rage. They can twist sorrow from the very marrow of our bones. They chew on us, spit us out, and leave us spent. But after we have given ourselves to grief and are ready to move on, the angel of gratitude will take us by the hand, lift us to our feet, inject energy into our weary hearts, and blanket us with a warm calm. Gratitude, in my mind, is synonymous with mercy.

When I recite what I appreciate in my life, the list grows by itself: my husband's humor and the depth of his devotion; my son's tenderness, peace, and ability to make me laugh; my daughter's affection, sharp mind, and the bold chances she takes as she defines herself; the whites beneath my dog's brown eyes, the purr that hums from my cat; my colleagues at work; my job; what I do in my job; the picture window in my living room; the view outside the window; my sauna; the mileage I get in my car; how well it drives; my smart, funny, creative, and loving community of friends; that I have ample food; that I am safe; that I live in America where we can differ politically and go to the same parties without killing each other. And yoga.

Giving attention to all the good that inhabits our lives somehow, miraculously, brings about more good. I believe it's one of the best-kept secrets of the universe.

I may not be able to go into certain hip poses at yoga class, but I absolutely have learned how to soar with appreciation.

Choices are the hinges of destiny.
PYTHAGORAS

HELEN'S STORY

Opportunity is missed by most people, because it is dressed in overalls and looks like work.
THOMAS EDISON

After Helen was diagnosed with lymphoma in 1982, her doctors told her that she might have six months left to live or she might have twenty-two years.

"I took the twenty-two years," she said, with a lilt in her voice. "When most people are given a prognosis, they believe whatever they're told. The issue for me was, 'Am I ready to face my own death?'"

The answer would unfold in the coming years. But first things first, and that meant completing two years of chemotherapy. The best part of her treatment, she says, was that she didn't like her oncologist.

"I find that when people like their doctors, they get sicker. I didn't like seeing my oncologist, but I swore to myself that I'd participate in anything that had to do with healing. Because of that, I joined a group called I Can Cope. Over six weeks, they asked us to look at our nutrition, our mobility, what would become of our worldly goods, which cemetery we wanted to be buried in—things like that. It was tough, but for me, it began the process of facing death."

When her two years of chemo were complete, Helen began working with a counselor who was also a massage therapist. Her healing technique was to talk with the patient about emotional wounds while simultaneously working on the body. It was transformational for Helen.

"With her help, I managed to see that the cancer was a sign that my life was going wrong. I wasn't making the kinds of decisions that I needed to make for my own health. The chemo had broken down my body; I was sharing a house with my ex-husband, and I needed to completely revamp my life. Although, my oncologist advised against it, I decided to move to California."

Helen also began working with different spiritual counselors to help her exhume the emotional skeletons that tripped her up, and she joined a woman's group at her church. She finally had the self-esteem to start her new life, and she was able to establish a new foundation.

"I realized there were other things available to me, that I didn't have to accept Western medicine. But I played both sides of the fence for a while. I visited an expert in lymphoma at Stanford. The tumors were still there, but they weren't growing. The doctor assumed the attitude of 'benign neglect.' That means they don't do anything about it; they just watch. If things change, they act."

"Living with cancer is harder than dying from it," Helen claimed. "Every headache you get you think is a brain tumor. You have to beat back the fear."

Continuing her spiritual practice gave her strength. She received a laying on of hands at Grace Cathedral in San Francisco. She joined in a healing ceremony in San Jose. She visited an ashram at Mount Madonna. She began taking herbs, and she consulted with an Ayurvedic doctor. All of this contributed to the peace that a very healthy, seventy-six-year-old Helen experiences today.

"The emotional journey I took brought me to the point of looking death straight on. The key is to face death. We assume it's painful, and for some, it may be. There can be a lot of fear, but there are other ways of dying, too. There are ceremonies to release the soul. You have to look at the *process* of dying. It's about leaving structures behind. The ego is what gives us the most pain about death. Once you face that the ego is what makes you struggle, you can give it up. Once you release the ego, you can reunite with the greater consciousness. You can stand back and admit that who you are *is* that greater consciousness."

Helen now works with dying patients at a hospice. She has learned that in this environment, people are given the choice to live or die, and very often the ones who die are missing a purpose, don't feel that they need anything, or don't feel needed by others.

"I have a friend with esophageal cancer," Helen reported. "She's bound and determined not to let the doctors have the last say. She was sent to hospice after just one round of chemo, but when she got the idea that she needed to get a book published, things changed. She got up and drove home." Helen told me that facing death is the one thing that frees you.

Helen's commitment to spiritual work suggests that she has a deep and unshakable faith. She doesn't see it that way. "I'm very much the pragmatist. What works, works. That's why I've gone through all the stuff I've gone through. I went from yoga to meditation to whatever. It didn't matter. The approach I took made me vigilant, very watchful. Does this tea help? Does that kind of herb make a difference? I paid close attention to how I felt when I did everything and anything. Watchfulness is healing. It's taking back power, a power that has the capacity to save people." The downside, Helen admitted, is that "sometimes you can feel guilty that you got cancer in the first place."

Although Helen no longer monitors her disease through medical doctors, she believes she's fundamentally healed.

She reiterated her belief that an emotional state of mind was at the root of why she got the disease. "I gave all my control away when I got married. It was all my own doing. Giving away my power was the most destructive thing I've ever done in my life. Women have a responsibility to stand up for themselves. We shouldn't give our control over to anyone, ever. That includes being financially independent."

As part of taking control of her life, Helen promised herself that she would spend her fifty-fifth birthday on a beach. She wanted to go on a cruise around the Mediterranean. She dreamed of being a great artist. She eventually accomplished all of these things, plus she sailed across the ocean over stormy seas as part of a three-member crew. It was her proudest moment.

"When you have cancer, you have to change your life—bit by bit by bit. Change your diet. Change your friends. Change your profession. Change your living quarters. Change the things that don't work for you, and one by one, you'll see what happens."

These days, good things are still happening for Helen. Years ago someone told her that she would make a good editor and that she ought to think about running a publishing company. She just recently received her license to do business.

"I won't stop until I do this," she affirmed. "It's just the next thing."

We each need to let our intuition guide us, and then be willing to follow that guidance directly and fearlessly.
SHAKTI GAWAIN

MARCIA PRENGUBER, ND, FABNO

Goshen Center for Cancer Care

Everything you are against weakens you.
Everything you are for empowers you.
DR. WAYNE DYER

"Integrative care is the future in cancer care," said Dr. Marcia Prenguber, a naturopathic practitioner who is the director of integrative care and natural medicine at the Goshen Center for Cancer Care. "People have been so disenfranchised by being told, 'This is what you have to do, end of discussion, no matter what the side effects,' that they're flocking to alternative options. But it's hard to figure out what's legitimate in the alternative world. There are a lot of people out there who just want to make money, but there are also those who are doing significant and effective work."

Making money is nothing new when it comes to treating cancer, but blending both allopathic and complementary treatments *is* new, relatively speaking at least. This integrative approach isn't mainstream yet, but it's catching on in larger hospitals. And smaller, independent centers are cropping up everywhere.

To Dr. Prenguber, it simply makes sense. "People are more comfortable supporting their bodies while pouring chemotherapy into their systems. The benefit is that when the two are combined, the individual can carry on a good quality of life."

An example of how differently people are treated at the nonprofit Goshen Center compared to a strictly allopathic hospital would go something like this: at an allopathic hospital, a woman with breast cancer would be evaluated and then undergo a lumpectomy, which would be followed by radiation. At Goshen, she has a choice of what type of radiation therapy to have. Brachytherapy is a procedure in which a catheter is placed into the area where the tumor was removed. A radiation balloon inside the catheter targets the affected area, because the entire breast does not necessarily need radiation. Treatment is twice a day for five days. (It is appropriate only for specific types of breast cancer.)

During treatment, she meets with a naturopathic physician, a dietitian, and a counselor in order to discuss other aspects of her health care. The topics cover a range of things that affect health and reduce the risk of cancer recurrence. The counselor may help her learn how to cope with this new diagnosis, address the mental and emotional effects of treatment, and help family members understand how to support her. The dietitians will review what foods are best to keep in her diet on a regular basis, which foods to avoid while going through treatment, and what activities may be inappropriate given her specific diagnosis.

At the same time that radiation and chemo are being administered, naturopathic remedies can help heal wounds, relieve burning, and mitigate other side effects. These include natural therapies such as vitamins and herbal formulas. In addition, naturopathic oncologists will review supplements that should be avoided during the treatment.

Tumors need blood flow to survive and spread. The process of creating blood vessels that feed cancer is called "angiogenesis."

"Specific actions within the tumor call the blood supply to it," explained Dr. Prenguber. "The process of anti-angiogenesis is when you stop the blood supply from getting to the tumor. There are some pharmaceutical drugs that can accomplish this, but we're also finding that several foods have this capability."

Natural Remedies for Anti-Angiogenesis

Pharmaceutical companies have invested big bucks in the research and development of anti-angiogenic drugs. They've had some luck, and that's hopeful.

The irony, of course, is that the drug companies are attempting to mimic the compounds found in many foods and herbs that are anti-angiogenic by nature. We could wait until drug companies develop a magic bullet, then pay top dollar to take it, or we can go the local health-food store and incorporate these foods into a regular diet. When you see the list, you'll realize how easy it will be to do that. Personally, I like the part about having a glass of red wine as part of my treatment!

Since the research isn't conclusive yet, we don't know how much of these compounds are necessary in order to create effective panaceas. Meanwhile, it won't hurt to start incorporating these things into your diet. Obviously, you're not going to go out and buy a snake for its venom or chew the bark off the tree in your front yard. But you can certainly start cooking with the spices and consider supplementing your diet with the other items.

Here's a list of some of the natural products currently being researched for their anti-angiogenic properties:

- Curcumin (found in turmeric)
- Garlic
- Ginseng
- Green tea
- Licorice
- Mushrooms and other fungi
- Omega-3 and omega-6 fatty acids
- Quercetin
- Red wine
- Shark cartilage
- Snake venom
- Soybeans
- THC (tetrahyrocannabinol)
- Tree bark
- Vitamin D3

For more information, go to the Angiogenesis Foundation, angio.org.

Extracts from anti-angiogenesis foods and cruciferous vegetables have been created in capsule form, but as of yet, there are no studies to determine if they are as effective as chowing down on the real food.

"While there are a number of studies on many natural therapies, more are needed," Dr. Prengruber said. "Many large cancer centers advise patients to avoid natural therapies. Without the expertise of practitioners such as naturopathic physicians, who have been trained in the use of natural therapies and herb-drug-nutrient interactions, that's not such a bad decision. The potential for good with the use of these therapies is great, but without the training to evaluate the effects and interactions, there remains potential for harm."

Whether there is extensive research to back up the empirical evidence or not, it's clear that both nutrition and natural supplements play a big part in integrative therapy. "If someone has severe nausea and immune deficiency because of their chemo, we have a dietician on staff who can educate the patient about the foods that will work best for them. Even if someone has a good diet, they may not know which foods will support them the most once they start chemo."

The guiding principle behind Goshen's philosophy is teamwork. "Everyone works together," Dr. Prenguber said. "The oncologist tells the naturopath what approach he or she is taking. Then the naturopath meets with the patient to determine what to do to minimize side effects and enhance the effect of the treatment. We also help the patient learn what to do on a long-term basis to improve lifestyle habits and reduce the risk of recurrence."

When asked about the mind-body connection, Dr. Prenguber emphasized that the relationship between the mind and the body is demonstrated every day. "We tend to see it in negative ways. For example, if you're worried, you can't sleep. If you're anxious, your blood pressure goes up or blood sugars become out of balance. But we can help patients to turn that negative relationship around and make it a positive one." Dr. Prenguber explained there are good reasons to do this. "We find that when a patient decides to participate in his or her own treatment, there's a big difference in outcomes and overall well-being."

Goshen provides counselors who teach patients breathing, relaxation, and calming techniques, as well as creative visualization. Dr. Prenguber said this particular aspect of integrative care has been especially helpful for those undergoing radiation with neck or head cancers. Many have to wear a molded mask, and their movement is inhibited during the procedure, which can create extreme anxiety in some people. Relaxation techniques help, not only during radiation treatments, but also long after. "They see what effect a positive approach has on them personally. These are the same patients who tell me that cancer was the best thing that ever happened to them. That doesn't necessarily mean they're cured, but they experience the cancer in a healing way."

Given this holistic approach to healing, it seems illogical that every hospital in the U.S. isn't doing the same thing. Apparently, it comes down to research and money. According to Dr. Prenguber, since natural substances can't be patented, nobody wants to put research dollars into them. "The public has expressed its desire for more alternatives," she said. "There are also professionals who want to treat cancer this way, so we need to create a new paradigm to figure out the bigger picture. We need to broaden our thinking about how to evaluate the effectiveness of common nutrition, and push harder for studies on natural approaches to healing. It will probably have to come from government funding, though, because private industry won't do it."

Meanwhile, Dr. Prenguber is grateful for the integrative options available at Goshen. "The patients love our approach. I see changed people. They're very appreciative of a team working together for their well-being."

The Particulars

Where: Goshen, Indiana, about 120 miles southeast of Chicago and 150 miles north of Indianapolis.

Who: 4 medical oncologists;
2 radiation oncologists;

2 surgical oncologists and 1 breast surgeon;

3 naturopathic physicians, 1 of whom is also an acupuncturist;

2 registered dietitians; and

2 psychoneuroimmunology (PNI) counselors

Dr. Prenguber says, "We have a fabulous staff of nurses and other patient-focused support staff. We are a magnet hospital—that says a lot about our nursing staff!

"We have visionary leadership in the Goshen Health System CEO and the cancer center leadership. They are very clear on the role of the patient and that what we need to do is meet the needs of the patient."

What to expect: Patient records are requested for appointments at the Goshen Center for Cancer Care. Patients may self-refer or be referred by their family doctor. When the appointments are set up, records are requested to arrive before the patients' appointments. Patients meet with the surgical, medical, and/or radiation oncologist and with a naturopathic physician. Within five days, they are also scheduled to meet with one of the cancer center's registered dietitians and with one of the psychoneuroimmunology (PNI) counselors. The counselors help the patients to understand the relationship of the mind and the body, and how the patients can participate in their own healing process. Once patients have met with the physicians, any further evaluation, in the form of scans, X-rays, biopsies, blood work, and so on, is ordered before a treatment plan is developed.

Where to stay: If patients come from a distance, they have the opportunity to stay at the CARE House.

This homelike facility was built expressly to accommodate a patient and their caregiver during multiple-day treatments. There are four suites available, plus a large kitchen in which they can prepare and enjoy their meals, and a living room with a TV for entertainment. This is provided at no cost, and donations are welcome.

Cost: The cost for the medical, surgical, and radiation services at the Goshen Center for Cancer Care parallel what they are elsewhere. The services of the naturopathic physicians, the dietitians, and the counselors are provided at no additional cost.

Words of wisdom: "This approach to cancer care," said Dr. Prenguber, "is obviously so much more patient focused, caring, and supportive; how is it that every clinic is not doing this? I am asked how we manage it financially, and the answer is salaried physicians. The patient is the center with an integrative team of physicians and other health care practitioners. The model allows us to use a variety of services to address patient care without burdening the patient with extra expenses. It works."

Contact Information:

Goshen Center for Cancer Care
200 High Park Avenue
Goshen, Indiana 46526
866-496-HOPE
cancer.goshenhealth.org

Concentrate all your thoughts upon the work at hand. The sun's rays do not burn until brought to a focus.
ALEXANDER GRAHAM BELL

BARRY BOYD, MD, FACP

Changing the Cancer Culture

Author of *The Cancer Recovery Program: How to Increase the Effectiveness of Your Treatment and Live a Fuller, Healthier Life*

Keep away from people who try to belittle your ambitions. Small people always do that, but the really great

make you feel that you, too, can become great.
MARK TWAIN

Dr. Barry Boyd has been a practicing medical oncologist since 1993. In 1998, he founded the Integrative Medicine Program at Greenwich Hospital–Yale Health Systems, where he is currently the director of nutritional oncology. He is an assistant clinical professor, the director of curriculum in nutrition, and the director of curriculum of integrative medicine at Yale School of Medicine and an affiliate member of the Yale Cancer Center. He was also the associate clinical director of the Weill Cornell Center for Complementary and Integrative Medicine at New York Presbyterian Hospital.

Dr. Boyd obviously brings insights from alternative and integrative treatments to his practice, but he doesn't call himself an alternative doctor at all. Nor does he admit to working outside the box. "I call it a bigger box. I use conventional treatments in unconventional ways. In addition, much of what is scientifically valid, such as nutrition and lifestyle factors, has not been actively integrated into cancer care. These areas are within the bigger box!" he exclaimed enthusiastically.

It's reassuring (and inspires much needed hope) to know that there are MDs working within the traditional system who recognize the dysfunctional nature of how cancer is being treated and how cancer patients may be subject to what he calls "medical hexing."

"The nocebo effect is the opposite of the placebo effect," Dr. Boyd explained. "If a doctor tells a patient their outcome will be bad, then ... people are susceptible. Their outcome probably will be bad. But that's not just a function of biology; it's also the result of giving up because you think there is no hope."

Dr. Boyd recalled a patient who was diagnosed with the early stages of lung cancer. "The man had an early but very treatable pneumonia. I knew we could treat him, and he'd be OK. I admitted him to the hospital on Friday, signed him out to a colleague, and when I returned on Monday, I found that he had died. I asked the family what had happened. They said that the covering doctor had said to the patient, 'I am sorry you have terminal cancer.' At that point, they said the patient just gave up. He quickly declined and died the next morning. The family was sure it was the devastating impact of those words. He had been 'hexed.'"

In 1994, Dr. Boyd founded and became director of the integrative medicine program at Greenwich Hospital–Yale New Haven Health, and in 2000, he opened the Boyd Center for Integrative Health, which is devoted to cancer, nutrition, and lifestyle. He has worked with the Connecticut Challenge, a cancer-survivor charitable organization based at Yale, in order to develop a model cancer survivorship program within the Boyd Center.

Dr. Boyd believes that instilling hope in newly diagnosed cancer patients is not only important, but also realistic. "I believe in what I call the Mutual Fund Rule, which states that past performance is no guarantee of future results. In cancer treatment, past prognostic data is not an indication of future outcomes, even though patients are frequently given a prognosis that can only be derived from prior studies. I rarely give a specific prognosis based on statistics. I've had patients who have remained free of recurrence and off treatment for years with a number of different advanced cancers, often with dire prognoses at the time of diagnosis. You can change your biology, in part by how you feel. I'm convinced of that."

By the sound of it, you'd think the mind-body relationship is where Dr. Boyd focuses his medical attention, but providing hope and bypassing the nocebo effect is simply the platform of his work. His true passion is rooted in the science and study of what causes and cures cancer.

In our conversation, Dr. Boyd, who was so excited by his passion for the subject, talked so fast and rattled off so many university studies that my fingers couldn't keep up. What I gleaned from the conversation is that Dr. Boyd believes that the existing paradigm of cancer treatment must be reformatted, starting with what goes on inside medical schools. Specifically, they need to integrate nutrition, exercise, and lifestyle into the curriculum and determine how they can either lower the risk of getting cancer or help cure it.

"Oncology is driven by pharmaceutical drugs, and medical students are taught to rely on them. But if you can increase the survival rate of cancer by up to 40 or 50 percent with lifestyle changes alone, shouldn't we be teaching that?"

Dr. Boyd then referred to a study that questioned medical students about how they perceive the role of nutrition when treating cancer.[1] "In their first year of med school, they thought nutrition was of value. But each year, the value they placed on it progressively decreased until, by the time they graduated, they thought nutrition was of limited value. This was particularly true of students planning to become specialists (which is, by now, the majority of medical school graduates) rather than primary-care physicians. It gets trained out of them. Nutrition never gets coherently understood as a vital role in people's health, so essentially they ignore it."

Dr. Boyd then elaborated on how deeply embedded prescription drugs are in the medical culture, even if dietary changes work as well or better. "Studies in the 1980s suggested that women in countries where low-fat diets are prevalent are less inclined to get breast cancer.[2] This led to theories that both risk and survival from breast cancer can be influenced by dietary fat intake.[3,4] While the role of dietary fat and risk remains unclear, in 2006 the Women's Intervention Nutrition Study study reported on the effect of low dietary fat (20 percent) on breast cancer outcomes. The investigators found that low fat intake resulted in fewer recurrences and lower mortality. This was particularly true in women who had estrogen-nonresponsive cancers, a group that has a particularly unfavorable risk for recurrence.[5] This was hugely important.

"After a seven-year study of American women, it was concluded that this low-fat diet seemed to make a big difference. But that same year, a breast cancer drug called Herceptin came out. Both the drug and low-fat diet data were presented at the same meeting, but the uproar and excitement about the Herceptin data was dramatic,[6] while the low-fat study garnered limited interest among the attendees. This was even though the data on the nutritional study showed more success in the estrogen-nonresponsive women than the Herceptin did in the HER2-positive women.

"The bottom line is this: if you're talking about lifestyle change, whether it's through exercise or nutrition, it's not going to make money for anyone, including doctors. Perhaps more importantly, if physicians don't understand the biology of nutrition and lifestyle, they can't imagine how it can be as effective as a pharmacologic agent. They just don't believe the data. It's a failure of education and, more importantly, imagination!

"Unfortunately, in large studies of cancer survivors by the American Cancer Society, only 5 percent follow lifestyle guidelines on exercise, diet, and smoking cessation.[7] The one change that's been uniformly successful is smoking cessation. It is worth noting that Medicare, Medicaid, and insurance companies pay doctors to counsel their patients to quit smoking, but that's it. They don't do the same for talking about diet or exercise. That's too bad because, for instance, in the case of colorectal cancer, if you initiate exercise just six to eight hours a week, you have a 50 percent less chance of recurrence—just from walking."

Dr. Boyd has a degree in nutritional biochemistry from the Institute of Human Nutrition at Columbia University, so the man knows what he's talking about. But that doesn't mean he bows to nutritional supplements as the answer to all our cancer woes. "There are potential risks with unsupervised supplement use. I also think they should be more closely monitored and possibly regulated. Betacarotene is a good example," he continued. "In the 1960s and '70s it became clear that smoking was associated with lung cancer. There were studies that showed that when people ate more vegetables and fruits, they had less incidence of lung cancer, and many studies identified betacarotene as the critical nutrient.[8,9,10] It was also recognized as generally safe, even in high doses, with the exception of the orange hue imparted to the skin. Many smokers began taking betacarotene, often at the urging of their physicians or alternative practitioners.

"That gave a good glow to the supplement, but then in the 1990s, a US National Cancer Institute–sponsored critical study (called ATBC) of Finnish male smokers showed that smokers who were given vitamin E or betacarotene had an 18 percent higher risk of getting lung cancer with the betacarotene.[11] A year later, an American study, called CARET, showed that people have a 28 percent greater chance of getting the disease if they smoked and took betacarotene.[12]

"It changed our whole understanding of single nutrients. Unfortunately, while recognized by cancer-prevention specialists as a pivotal study in our understanding of single nutrients and cancer risk, it has virtually disappeared from the public's (and most MDs') screen. In the study on nutrient use among cancer patients, only 4 of over

250 patients taking multiple nutrients were even aware of this downside to betacarotene. If you go to any health-food store, you can find sources of supplemental betacarotene, but the clerks are totally unaware of this risk. And there is no warning label on the bottle!"

Plus, popping pills—even vitamins, minerals, and herbs—isn't the answer, according to Dr. Boyd. "Supplements are often necessary in the face of inadequate diet or frank deficiency, or periods of increased need, such as in the elderly or folate for pregnant women. Eating the right foods is far more important than taking nutritional supplements. People just need to eat better."

One important exception, said Dr. Boyd, is vitamin D. Because of our modern lifestyle, vitamin D is deficient in a large segment of the population. He says that this is the one nutrient where supplementation is critical for everything from bone health to cardiovascular and diabetic risk to cancer risk and survival. However, like every nutrient, even vitamin D has a safe upper limit.

In addition, Dr. Boyd is concerned that the money being made by practitioners in alternative circles who rely heavily on supplements may bias their views on risk and benefit. "I'm very nervous about people who are making lots of money from treating diseases with nutraceuticals that have been inadequately tested for both benefit and risk. You have to be careful of these businesses that have been contaminated by financial interests. Unfortunately, I see new patients in my office daily who sometimes spend thousands of dollars a month on supplements in hopes of attaining a cure. We must be careful what we promise patients with these approaches, because patients are extremely vulnerable and willing to do almost anything to get better. I believe that, as physicians, we have a special obligation to truly understand the risk and potential value of integrative therapies."

Billion-dollar pharmaceutical companies take the lead when it comes to profiting from illness. Given that making money is their goal, I asked Dr. Boyd how to square the need for true advances in cancer treatment while being under the financial fist of the drug companies. "We need people who are devoted to finding answers to what contributes to cancer and how we can regain good health. It's happening slowly. But there are now some exciting results surfacing from studies about food, natural substances, and the overall environment of the body in relation to cancer."

Two studies in particular are of interest to Dr. Boyd. One study from the H. Lee Moffit Cancer Center in Tampa, Florida, published in April 2009, scientifically supports what practitioners in alternative circles have been purporting for years: that the pH balance in the body is important.[13] The more acidic the body chemistry, the more rapidly a tumor will grow. The more alkaline, the slower the tumor will grow, or it will stop growing altogether. The study demonstrated that an alkaline environment reduced both invasiveness and spread of malignancy. Hopefully, maintaining a good pH balance will soon become a standard recommendation for cancer patients.

The next finding is good—no, *great*—news for coffee lovers: in a series of studies at the University of Oslo in Norway, researchers assessed the chief source of dietary antioxidants.[14] Surprisingly, among Norwegians, over 60 percent came from coffee, while tea contributed 8 percent, berries 13 percent, and vegetables 4 percent.

This finding is hardly surprising to Dr. Boyd. "We are only beginning to truly study foods rather than individual nutrients. It also reflects recent evidence that coffee has many health benefits, including reduced risk of diabetes, Parkinson's disease, cirrhosis, chronic liver disease, and even some cancers. Tea has often attained mythic status as a 'magical food,' while coffee has been seen simply as a vehicle for caffeine. Yet it is richly endowed with a variety of valuable phytonutrients."

Coffee drinkers who think green tea is wimpy can rejoice. But, said Dr. Boyd, doctors may not pay much attention to the data. "The way to teach doctors about the relationship between food and cancer has to be scientific. If we can explain the mechanism of how diet and exercise can change the biology of cancer, they'll listen. They don't like to talk about nutrition because it's not sexy, but they do like to talk about molecular biology."

The impact of food is just one piece of the cancer puzzle that Dr. Boyd is scrutinizing. He's also intrigued by this fact: humans, domestic animals, and zoo animals have the highest incidence of cancer on the planet. Why?

"Throughout history, both animals and man have had periods of involuntary limitation in caloric availability. Virtually every organism has had to cope with periods of low food availability, in addition to other environmental stresses, and as a result has evolved complex molecular responses to these events. The result is a reduction in the rate of cell growth, decline in glucose and insulin levels, and a reduction in reproductive ability—exactly what you need during periods of famine.

"Unfortunately, we now have consistent availability of high-calorie foods without the need to expend calories to get them (unlike our forebears), which isn't natural. It's built into our biology that we would benefit from fasting every now and then. To me, it makes sense that we—and our domestic and zoo animals—should limit calories periodically.

"One approach is so-called alternate-day modified fasts, which reduce calories to a minimum every other day while allowing a normal intake of calories on the other days. This appears to induce the same series of genetic programs that have worked in our favor for millions of years and that occur with long-term calorie limitation. It is just far easier to know the next day you don't have to limit your intake.

"Several studies sponsored by the National Institutes of Health are being conducted to explore this new theory.[15] We are developing an alternate-day modified fast for cancer survivors who are overweight in order to explore the potential health benefits and the feasibility for longer term fasts, in which the fasting is done once or twice per week.

"And that's just the tip of the iceberg. There are all kinds of things we're looking at," he said. "Height and weight are important. These reflect very early, often prenatal exposures to toxins, not just adult lifestyle. In addition, people have been exposed over the last fifty years to an increasing burden of pesticides, and our bodies contain varying levels of pesticides in adipose stores. A series of studies from a large national program called the National Health and Nutrition Examination Survey (NHANES) looked at weight, pesticide levels, and diabetes risk.[16] For example, increasing levels of pesticides tended to create a greater risk of diabetes. Those who were very heavy, but had low pesticide levels, had no diabetic risk. This suggests that the stored pesticides in the fat may be triggering the diabetes.

"It's also important to look at *when* people are exposed to pesticides. A study from California showed that adult women who, at age fourteen or younger, had high blood levels of organochlorine pesticides had five times the incidence of breast cancer in their fifties and older than those who had low levels at age fourteen and younger.[17] Previous studies, including the Long Island Breast Cancer Study Project (LIBCSP), failed to show a link between pesticide levels and breast cancer risk, but they looked at levels drawn and measured at diagnosis rather than earlier years in childhood."[18]

Dr. Boyd said that this newer understanding of the connection between earlier exposures and the risk of later adult disease doesn't necessarily coincide with women's own perception of why they got the disease. A study was published in 2006 on women's understanding of breast cancer. Dr. Boyd reports: "Most women thought genetics were the leading cause of breast cancer. They overestimated the genetic risk as over 50 percent, while it's actually only about 15 percent. In their view, the second leading cause was from smoking. While smoking is the leading cause of lung cancer and several other cancers, there's really not that much evidence of a connection with breast cancer. Finally, they considered pollution and pesticides, which are the two largest risk factors related to reproductive and other hormonal factors, such as ages of first period and menopause, ages of first full-term pregnancy, breast feeding, and so on. Despite their important role in the rise in breast cancer incidence over the last thirty years, pollution and pesticides were ranked lowest in perceived risk."[19]

Obviously, perception poses yet another set of variables when considering how and why we get cancer. Dr. Boyd understands clearly the relationship between our thoughts and physiology. He cited the breakthrough work in the science of psychoneuroimmunology. "In a way, it's simple. When you're under stress, the adrenal gland releases stress hormones, such as cortisol and epinephrine. If the stress is chronic, this results in increased weight gain, particularly in the mid-abdomen, a so-called visceral obesity. This leads to increasing levels of insulin and related growth factors, which have been shown to enhance cell growth and worsen outcome in a number of cancers. If you reduce stress, in addition maintaining a sound exercise and nutrition program, high levels of insulin can be suppressed, the speed of tumor growth can be reduced, and cancer survival rates can be potentially and significantly changed for the better. This relationship is central to understanding the biology of how diet and lifestyle can improve cancer survival."

In Dr. Boyd's world, there's a lot to hope for, but he understands how common it is for cancer patients to lose hope after visiting their local cancer center. "The problem with some institutions is that they tell you there's nothing left to do. They leave little room for hope. But what they may be saying is that there's nothing available at *their* institution, that they have run out of protocols at *their* institution. That's when you just have to walk out the door and look for another open door."

Contact Information:

15 Valley Drive
Greenwich, CT 06830
medingen.com/advisoryBoard_boyd.htm

*Hope is not a dream, but a way of
making dreams become reality.*
CARDINAL LEON JOSEPH SUENENS

CHAPTER 8

Intuition

It is the heart, always, that sees before the head can see.
THOMAS CARLYLE

There's nothing wrong with logic and reason, but intuition is a completely different animal and one that can't be ignored. To heal, we need a lot of ingredients: authority, forgiveness, trust, courage, and conviction. But intuition, if we exercise its gifts, will take us closer to ourselves and reveal more about our inner truth and the universe that supports us. I believe intuition is a vital God-given power, the channel through which our souls (and other invisible forces) attempt to guide us.

One of the blessings about my cancer diagnosis (other than the fact that it improved my life by leaps and bounds) is that it sharpened my senses and my receptivity. After the third diagnosis, I was on high alert. The doctors didn't have much to offer, and

I had an awful lot to lose. Every cell in my body was wide open to receiving pathways of recovery. I was more watchful than ever before, more aware and more tuned in to signs of the nonphysical support that is always here, but not often recognized.

That's our biology at work when we're freaked out. Unlike a shot of adrenalin after an earthquake or a car accident, living in an intuitive state is truly an altered state of consciousness that can manifest from crisis. Given that a diagnosis is a long-term situation, senses may be heightened for months at a time rather than the minutes or hours after an immediate emergency. This long-term alertness sets up the perfect environment for intuiting the world around us.

According to medical intuitive Laura Alden Kamm, intuition expresses itself through physical sensations.[1] Some people feel it, others hear it, and still others have visions. After my first two diagnoses, intuition came to me through auditory channels. I clearly heard, "It's OK. You'll be all right." It took a while, but as it turns out, I really am all right.

Many people reading this book probably already have a working relationship with intuition. If you're not one of those but would like to be, just move a little slower when making decisions. As an option presents itself to you, spend a moment paying full attention to your body as it absorbs the atmosphere of that choice. Then take that time with the next option, and the next. If you notice something different about your reaction to one option, discern what it means. Identify how your intuition is speaking to you. Do you hear something? Feel something? See something? Intuition is also a great guide after you've asked the universe for something specific.

After my third diagnosis, I put out an all-points bulletin to all nonphysical beings, asking them to reassure me that the choices I was making (raw foods, alternative doctors, writing this book) were right for me. I became hyper-receptive, and I invited my intuition to point things out to me that I might not otherwise see. In a single day, I found supportive answers all over the place. I was out of town and needed a haircut, so I drove around an upscale retail area and came upon a place called Oxygen Salon & Spa. Cancer doesn't like oxygen, so I decided it was a good choice and went in. Typically, they didn't have openings for walk-ins, but that day they did. The stylist assigned to me was studying to become a nutritional healer—the very path I was choosing for my treatment. I took that as a very good sign.

On that same trip, I intuitively brought my tennis racquet with me, even though I was traveling solo. The same day that I got my hair cut, I drove by a public tennis club I had never seen before, despite the fact that I had driven that same road hundreds of times. I slammed some balls against the backboard, then rented a cheap ball machine so I could work out some of my anxiety. Without listening to my intuition, I wouldn't have brought my racquet. Without paying attention, I wouldn't have noticed the courts. Later that same day, I saw a sign posted on a door that read: *Your Future Is Certain and Good. Have Faith.* And I do.

A few weeks later, I took Kamm's book, *Intuitive Wellness,* to read during my lunch hour. I wanted to be outside, but the sun was too hot, and a shaded park was too far away. I figured I'd go to a nearby café, when I flashed on a subdivision my mother had lived in about a decade before. It was close by, and I recalled that it had little ponds and big shade trees; I imagined a bench beneath a tree where I could read. I let my intuition guide me into an entrance and then kept allowing it to show me where to park. I found a place that felt right, and it turns out it was near a path that I had never seen before. I followed the path down to a small pond, and to my delight, a bench was perched beneath a tree awaiting my arrival. I had never been to this pond before.

These are small examples, but they're significant. When we habitually turn to our intuition for answers on the little things, we know we can trust it on the big stuff.

After my third diagnosis, when my sister told me about a woman with metastasized brain cancer who, among other things, started eating raw foods and is now cancer free, my intuition erupted. I felt as though something inside my body had landed elegantly into the right space. It was as if until then, a round peg within me had found only square holes. At last there was a fit. It was a very clear sensation.

Of course, it's smart to take some logical steps when deciding which doctor to work with, what kind of treatment to follow, when enough is enough, or who to include in your most intimate moments. But remember that your intuition is not of this world; it comes from a place of expanded understanding. It can help you with all your decisions in ways that the logical mind lacks.

Trusting intuition requires trusting yourself and your innate authority. Taming your ego and analytical mind to sit, stay, and quit barking can be hard. Intuition is very quiet and has little chance of being heard if you don't kennel up your mind chatter. But it's well worth stopping the mind chatter to hear your intuitive voice.

It's easy to judge ourselves when intuition is wrong, but logical choices can be wrong, too. We're not always right, no matter what source we pull from. I've come to trust my intuitive self more than the egocentric, analytical part of me that tends to get way too caught up in irrelevant details and is much too attached to outcomes.

Read Kamm's book—or another that feels right—and you'll enter into a new, deeper, more loving relationship with yourself and the vast realm of nonphysical support that's available to all of us. To me, intuition is the means by which we receive answers to our prayers.

Instinct is the nose of the mind.
DELPHINE GAY DE GIRARDIN

BETH'S STORY

I always wondered why somebody doesn't do something about that. Then I realized I was somebody.
LILY TOMLIN

Beth lives high in the Rocky Mountains, but thin oxygen didn't keep her from smoking for fifty years. That said, neither cigarettes nor altitude prevented her from hanging out on local ski slopes and alpine hiking trails.

When Beth was sixty-six, she retired from a high-stress job and wanted to spend the fall away from the cold, windy, snowy weather. She gave herself a trip to Vietnam. While she was away, however, she developed a nasty cough. Rather than feeling invigorated when she returned home, she was upset about the cough, about not having a job—or, in her mind, a life—and about returning to the gloomy mountain weather. She decided to ignore the cough, but at the same time, she knew it was finally time to quit smoking.

Even after she relinquished all of her cigarettes to her son, including those that she'd hidden away, the cough persevered. A week later, Beth saw a doctor, who listened to her lungs and assured her that everything was fine. But she had a strong sense that she wasn't fine and asked for a chest X-ray just to be sure. The cough, coupled with intense nicotine withdrawals, was making her feel miserable. She said, "I figured that if I had to struggle this hard to quit smoking, then the cough should be gone. I wanted that X-ray to see what was going on."

Her instincts were right: the film revealed a mass on her right lung.

Two days later, she was at a regional hospital where the tests began. The first was a biopsy. After the procedure, Beth heard what was clearly not for her ears. "They gave me a mild sedative and must have thought I was asleep, but I wasn't. The lab tech came in and said to the radiologist, 'It's malignant.' I kept pretending to be asleep because I had to process the news internally before I could deal with anybody else."

Beth's good friend happened to be the head of the emergency department at the hospital where the biopsy was performed. When she was up and around, he informed her that things weren't looking good. She asked him if he would take over as her doctor. He agreed and immediately ordered both a CT scan and an MRI to be done that same day.

"By the end of the day, I was told that I had a mass on each lung. I was lucky because there wasn't evidence of cancer anywhere else. I stared at the X-rays of my body. They said I needed to see the oncologist next. I was in shock."

Beth returned home to her tight-knit mountain community, stressed and uncertain. "News travels fast in small towns, and everyone tends to know everyone's business. I called a friend in New York who had survived breast cancer, and she became my mentor. Her first piece of invaluable advice was not to tell anyone who didn't have to know. She explained that once you say the word 'cancer,' you're not you anymore; you become an object, a piece of concern. Everyone is so sorry. They all want to help, and they all have advice."

Beth was also evaluating her own response to the diagnosis: "We all have this internal written script that describes how we're supposed to behave around such news. It was hard not to tell people, but if I were to accidentally blurt it out, I knew that all of a sudden everyone would be saying, 'How are you feeling?' with a tone of voice that gives them away. *They think you're dying.* I became supersensitive to how people treated me, trying to discern who might know my secret."

Beth only shared her news with family members. Even so, she admits that she initially played into the standard script for a cancer patient. "The doctor comes in wearing a white coat, holding a thick folder, and says, 'I'm really sorry to tell you this...' Everyone knows how you're supposed to behave after that, and I was no exception.

"The day after the diagnosis I went crazy. I was no longer me; I *was* cancer. It was cold and gray, and the wind was blowing. I paced around my house feeling like a trapped animal. I was having extreme nicotine withdrawals, and I had cancer. My role in the prescribed script was to update my will, clean out the closets, and start making videos of myself so my grandchildren would know who I was after I was gone."

Beth had been a massage therapist for thirty years; she had worked with healers and helped other people heal themselves. Now it was her turn to be the patient, and it wasn't easy. She was unclear about how she should proceed. She began discussing her options with her sons and their wives (one, a medical doctor; the other, a nutritionist and yoga teacher). Her family rallied. Her daughter-in-law who was a doctor researched lung cancer treatments from the allopathic standpoint, while the other one suggested that with a change of diet and lifestyle, she could kick the cancer.

A few days later, Beth was flanked by family and greeted by donuts and cookies in the lobby of the oncologist's office. While she was having a PET scan, the oncologist spoke to her family. "It was very disjointed and awkward," recalled Beth. "By the time I had completed the PET scan, the appointment with the oncologist was over. My kids told me what the doctor had said while we ate pizza at a nearby restaurant."

The doctor's suggestion was that Beth immediately start taking the drug Tarceva. "As we drove home, I was reading about all the side effects of this stuff and what the statistics were. It said that 34 percent of Tarceva patients are still alive six months after taking it. Something snapped in me. *What the hell?* I'm supposed to take this drug that will compromise my life so that in six months I'll have a 34 percent chance of still being alive? NOT!" Then there was the expense: a daily dose of the drug cost $90, and Beth didn't have Medicare's drug plan.

"What saved me at that point was that my son and his wife were going to Cabo San Lucas for Thanksgiving. I wanted to go and just escape from it all." Two days later, they were in Mexico, on the nineteenth floor of a high-rise on the beach. Beth had a big balcony that overlooked the ocean. She recalled, "As soon as I got there, I started letting the whole cancer scene fade away. We had some beers and a great dinner. After that, I went back outside on the balcony. I was looking at the sky and the ocean, and I thought, 'I'm not going to have cancer, and I'm not going to die.' It was a very clear voice. I listened; it resonated. I held on to the thought, and it became mine.

"I said it to myself over and over again: 'I am not going to die.' It became my mantra.

"The next day I told my daughter-in-law, 'I'm not going to have cancer.' She responded with: 'Denial is the first stage of acceptance, Beth.' And I said, 'No, I'm not going to have this cancer.'

"I knew she had done a lot of medical research that she wanted to share with me. I knew we were expected to sit and talk about my options, but I suggested we go swimming instead. I never allowed the cancer conversation to happen on that trip because I was in a different space. I simply didn't want to fill my head with a lot of allopathic knowledge about cancer, medical options, or life expectancy. I never did read anything over the course of the next few months."

When she returned home, Beth continued with her mantra, but still wasn't prepared to cancel her next oncology appointment. Meanwhile, she contacted Amanda, an acupuncturist and energy healer she knew. Beth asked if Amanda would help cure her. Amanda agreed and added that she'd like to invite others to work on her as well. With Beth's blessing, Amanda said she would immediately begin remote healing work and suggested that Beth start taking C-Answer, a brown seaweed used extensively in Japan as a cancer treatment. Thus began Beth's healing journey.

When she next saw her oncologist, the results of the PET scan mimicked the X-rays and indicated that there were indeed two masses, one in each lung. The doctor urged Beth to start taking Tarceva, but she had already moved away from that option.

"I told the oncologist that I had to think about it and get on a Medicare plan first, but the truth was that I was resisting becoming a pill taker and playing the patient. Instead, I was becoming a risk taker and forsaking the script of 'patient.' I also told the oncologist that I wanted a second opinion, which was true, so I called Sloan Kettering in New York and was put on a waiting list for patients seeking second opinions. Then I returned to Mexico with my family."

After a few days of lying on the hot, sandy beach, ducking waves, and repeating her mantra, Beth realized that no one on the trip had even uttered the word "cancer." The only mention of it was when she told her sister-in-law, "I don't have to die, you know." She said it to remind herself and them that this was true. Time passed happily for her, drinking margaritas and being mindless.

One day, they rented a car to explore the small town of Troncones, not far from Zihuatanejo. "We were looking at real estate, which we often did, when I found a little *palapa* on the beach near a yoga center. It was the place I had dreamed of for years, and it was for sale! I figured that if I were going to die, I would die there. If I were going to get well, this would be the place to do it. I knew I had to be somewhere hot, where I could bake the stuff out of me, and the ocean had always been a place of healing for me. I was ready to make an offer on the house."

The real estate agent informed her that the house had been on the market for two years, but that the owner wouldn't ever let it go. So Beth wrote an e-mail to the owner that night, hoping for a response. There was none.

Soon after, Beth flew directly from Mexico to New York to see a renowned doctor whose specialty was lung cancer. Noting that she had a mass in each lung, the doctor inquired why only one biopsy had been performed. Beth didn't know, and the doctor replied with an odd mixture of arrogance and hope that he didn't see a pathway on the X-ray where the cancer had traveled from one lung to the other.

"There's a 97 percent chance that it's the same cancer in both lungs," the doctor told her. "If it's a different cancer in each lung, then you probably have stage 1 cancer; if it's in both, then you may have stage 4."

She needed that second biopsy, but it would be six more weeks before Sloan Kettering could perform it. She suggested going back home and having the biopsy done there, and the doctor agreed to the plan.

"I kept telling myself that I wasn't going to have cancer, and I wasn't going to die. At the same time, I had agreed to get another biopsy, I was taking the brown seaweed faithfully, and I was talking to Amanda often. Although I was listening to both the allopathic and the holistic practitioners, I felt no contradiction at the time. Maybe I needed the allopathic folks to confirm that my holistic efforts were paying off. After all, they had machines to tell you what was going on, and most of my family wanted a message from the machines."

A week later, Beth was back at her regional hospital undergoing a CT scan to determine the exact position of the tumor. After the first image was taken, the tech told her something was wrong with the film, so they did it again. They took a second picture, then a third. Finally, the radiologist came to her and said, "I don't know what to tell you, but the left mass is almost completely dissolved. There is nothing to biopsy. It's some kind of miracle. Congratulations!"

"I was in a really strange place then," Beth remembered. "I couldn't believe it and felt that I didn't deserve it. I hadn't imagined that the mass would go away so quickly. I was as taken aback as they were at the hospital. I was light-headed and weak. I sat in my car trying to get it through my head that the tumor was gone. Gradually, it sunk in. Then I felt guilty for not trusting completely. It was completely affirming. That's all I can say. I offered up lots of prayers of gratitude.

"One daughter-in-law said that it was great news, while the other wondered whether there had been some kind of medical mistake."

Sloan Kettering received the results from the Western hospital and informed Beth that she could have surgery to remove the mass from the other lung on December 26. Beth said, "After just being gifted a miracle, it seemed rude and inappropriate to rush into surgery."

Then another unexpected thing happened. The owner of the palapa in Mexico e-mailed and said she would love to sell the house to Beth. The house would soon be hers.

"All my kids were coming to my mountain home for the holidays, and they hadn't all been together for Christmas in about five years. Amanda, the healer, was also coming to town after Christmas, and we had scheduled five straight days of working together. I told the doctor at Sloan Kettering that I would have the surgery later."

"'Look,' he said, 'cancer grows quickly, so you ought to do this right now.'

"I said I wasn't ready, which was totally the truth. His nurse called me a few days later, and I had to tell her the same thing: I wasn't ready to have surgery.

"Amanda arrived shortly after Christmas, and we began our work on releasing the cancer. She told me that before this lifetime, I had made an agreement about how long I would live, and it would be to age sixty-seven.

"'The first thing you have to do is decide if you want to redo your commitment,' Amanda said. 'Do you want to live another twenty years?'

"I didn't have a fast-and-certain answer. It's pretty heavy to redo a commitment that you make from another lifetime. I knew it was going against some subconscious thing that was going on. A few months back, I had thought I was going to die. Now the idea of living another twenty years took some thinking. I had to think about why I'd made that contract in the first place and determine if I truly wanted to live another twenty years. My mind went spinning off again, but by our session the next day, I'd decided that I wanted those twenty years."

What ensued were three more days of intense ritual, including "going beyond the beyond" and asking permission to change the contract for this lifetime. "When the permission was given, we did all kinds of practices. The last day we focused on removing the actual tumor. We did a bunch of visualization work, and after awhile, I could actually see into my lung and see the tumor very clearly.

"'Now let's take it out,' Amanda said. We did. We pulled it about a foot away from my body.

"Then the most amazing image came to me. It was of a boy named Henry who had been a butler in a play I'd helped produce. He was standing in front of me holding a silver tray. We put the tumor on the tray, and he stood there clear as dawn. Amanda then said we needed to take the tumor off the tray, place it in a crystalline chamber, send it up to the beyond, and have it dissolve. I was able to do that clearly with her help.

"I walked out of my session with Amanda feeling as though the tumor had, indeed, gone to the beyond. But later that day I began the cursed thinking again. My allopathic mind kept saying, 'I might still have it,' then I'd catch myself and insist, 'No, I don't have cancer!' The debate went on. Still, that day with Amanda, I surrendered more than I ever had before, and I saw the cancer go away. That was my work with Amanda. I could not have done it without her."

After the holidays, Sloan Kettering called Beth again, urging her to schedule surgery. "At this point I came up with a wonderful plan to be *absolutely* over and done with cancer. I would spend the entire month of January in Mexico doing healing work, and at the end of the month I'd go to New York, have another CT scan, and be prepared to either have the surgery or not, depending on the results of the scan."

Acquiring the house in Mexico represented how Beth's life was morphing from what it had been to what it would become. "Once I decided to create good things in my life, good things just started coming to me."

The doctors who had attended to her case were playing out a different story. The doctor at Sloan Kettering blamed her hometown docs for an error, doubting that a second mass had ever existed. Her hometown doctors convened a meeting to review the evidence of the second tumor at the time of diagnosis, and determined, in the face of overwhelming evidence, that the mass had indeed existed. Sloan Kettering persisted in blaming the others for what it could not understand: a tumor that had vanished.

Fortunately, Beth was out of the line of fire. Instead she spent nearly three weeks at her house in Mexico, lying on the hot sand, chanting her mantra, doing breathing exercises, practicing yoga, and "drinking margaritas every night so that I wouldn't get too serious."

By the time she flew to New York and had the CT scan, the doctor blankly said, "I've canceled your surgery. It's all gone. What did you do? What happened?"

"All I could say was, 'Thank you for not doing the surgery if I didn't need it.' There was a bit of silence between us until I said, 'Maybe it's a miracle.'

"He looked directly at me and said, 'We don't deal with miracles at Sloan Kettering.' I felt like I was supposed to apologize. But there I was, in shaky disbelief. Everything I had done on a spiritual level had just been validated by the most famous hospital in America.

I then asked him what percentage of patients have this experience. He said, 'I wouldn't know. There is no follow-up on cases like this. That's not something we do.'

"He wasn't interested in my situation. He was baffled and threatened. Later, I met with the alternative-medicine team once, but they were underwhelmed. They didn't want to probe into the depths of my story. When I told them I had worked with a healer, they didn't ask what else I'd done. They didn't explore my path at all."

After the surgery was canceled, Beth called Amanda and shouted, "It's gone!"

The healer was calm. "I know it's gone. I'm glad you're on board."

Beth spent the rest of the weekend in New York, partying with family and friends. Yet even though she was spirited away by a great sense of celebration, Beth found the situation disorienting. "It really changed me. I totally rewrote my script. I stopped going to the dentist, stopped balancing my checkbook. I let go of little responsibilities and gave myself to a political campaign. I wanted to do something really righteous. Then I went back to Mexico for the rest of the winter and continued to do my healing work, including dealing with feelings like, 'It's gone, but for how long? Why is it gone? How can I have it stay gone?'"

Beth admitted that she still hasn't figured it all out. "The hardest part about going into my fourth year is to strike a balance between arrogance and fear. Whenever I get sloppy with my lifestyle, I think I'm inviting it back and that I must have an unconscious desire to die. I have to stop myself and remind myself to be gentle."

To support her health, Beth has cut back on sugar and eats only organic chicken, and she eats an abundance of kale and other greens. Her family hunts wild game, so she'll eat venison and elk when it's available; she enjoys wild salmon also and, on occasion, some organic beef. She still drinks alcohol, but doesn't smoke at all, and she no longer suffers from nicotine cravings. She does not have an exercise routine, but when she's in Mexico, she does yoga regularly. She likes to walk outdoors and spends winters in the warmth of the Southern Hemisphere.

"I'm a specialist in guilt, but I continue to go through positive changes. I'm lighter and easier than I was before. I haven't figured out how and why I want to share my story. I haven't ever done anything with it, like write a book. I kind of get tired of the whole thing. I just want to be a person."

Whether she writes a book or simply continues to split her time between the mountains and Mexico, Beth is positively certain about one thing: "You don't have to die, which doesn't mean you're totally in charge by any means."

Only those who will risk going too far can possibly find out how far one can go.
T.S. ELIOT

LAURA ALDEN KAMM

Author of *Intuitive Wellness: Using Your Body's Inner Wisdom to Heal*

Have the courage to follow your heart and intuition. They somehow already know what you truly want to become. Everything else is secondary.
STEVE JOBS

My conversation with Laura Alden Kamm was exhilarating. As a medical intuitive and author of the book *Intuitive Wellness,* Laura has the ability to see things most people don't and to teach others how to foster their inherent intuitive nature. She wasn't born with this gift, however. She endured a long, serious illness, which culminated in a near-death experience. When she recovered, she had lost some of her sight, but ironically, she had gained a clear intuitive vision.

The subject of cancer is complex, even to someone as skilled as she is. The "morphic field" of cancer is large and powerful and carries a lot of momentum with it. According to Laura, the first step to reclaiming your power in order to handle the challenges you're facing is to look within for guidance, which will bring you direction and peace of mind.

"When you're struck with a diagnosis such as cancer, your whole world instantly shatters," Laura said. "You cling to any external source of support you can find. Yet one of the greatest supports for kindness and nurturing is within you. People know that in theory, but it's hard to live it practically."

Laura acknowledged that some people are afraid of what they'll find if they go inside and that self-discovery can be frightening. "It's a very personal journey," she said. "Each individual has to create their own map that will move them toward healing. The thought of that can make them more afraid than they were before. They wonder, 'How do I go inside if I don't know myself?'

"The best way to support yourself in the process of getting to know who you really are—and to know what part of you either caused or supported the cause of the disease—is through meditation or contemplation. If you're new to meditation, look into audio programs featuring someone or some practice with which you resonate. It could be Christian, Buddhist, Sufi—whatever works for you. And when

I say 'works for you,' I mean that there has to be a resonance. Resonating with something is the key that will open the door for you."

Throughout our conversation, Laura referred to the importance of paying close attention to those things that resonate. Again, it's a totally subjective experience, but each person can know if what they are considering doing or choosing resonates with them by paying attention to how they feel. If it feels right, it's resonating. If it feels off somehow, then it's not in balance.

"You have to understand resonance. Your job is to find the place of resonance with all that you do. The opposite of resonance is dissonance. The nature of disease is dissonance. When you find resonance, dissonance begins to disappear. But it won't let go of you until you go within and look at it straight in the face. You can't just hope it will go away."

Laura suggested going within not just to find comfort, but also to face your fear and the disease. "A great start is simply to go in and just say hello to *you*. When you do, your body responds with surrender and sweetness, and the path is revealed. The more stillness you seek, the more inner dialogue you will achieve. Through this inner dialogue with your body, you will become privy to the unseen and discover and know more of yourself.

"The willingness to say hello to the self and to the disease is important. The disease is embedded in part of the body. You cannot ignore the fact that being honest and authentic in your heart brings on the power of healing. Simplicity is the closest path to truth. You don't need a costume to talk to God or to your soul.

"Once you go inside, you can start having conversations with your inner selves, meaning the multiple aspects within you—the wounded child, the magical child, the little professor, the healer, the master, the teacher, the controller, and the protector—all of you. The controller and protector have a lot to do with your healing. But the controller especially has a lot to do with creating the environment that sets up pathways to resistance. Resistance, then, creates dissonance."

Laura writes in her book that all diseases start in the electromagnetic field. Cancer specifically possesses an emotional intelligence that is fiercely independent and rebellious. The core issues of cancer relate to feelings of fear, deep sadness, and grief. The spiritual intelligence of cancer includes perceptions of being cut off from life, feeling unable to truly express one's uniqueness, and a tendency to hide one's true feelings.

"When you go inside to get to know your disease, it's important to look at what it was within you that may have rebelled. To answer that question, ask yourself: where have you left yourself behind? That's usually where you'll find the rebel."

"Does that mean that all cancers start with an emotional component," I asked, "even in cases where it's clearly related to a physical condition, such as lifelong smoking?"

Laura replied, "It shows up first in the electromagnetic field, but that doesn't mean the cause is solely emotional. If you've smoked your entire life, the disease still shows up in the electromagnetic field first. Or if you've lived in a place full of toxins, those toxins will show up in your field first. It manifests as a specific electromagnetic form of condensation that exemplifies the toxin to which you were exposed, either recently or in the distant past. But not only toxins reside in the electromagnetic field; everything shows up there. If you just took a trip and the experience changed your perspective, that will also show up. If you're choosing the same type of person over and over again in a series of dysfunctional relationships, that will show up. If you're eating junk food or really good and nourishing food, that shows up in the electromagnetic field. All things moving in and out of your life and your body appear in the electromagnetic field first and then the body, which is obviously matter and a denser structure.

"Emotional intelligence is attached to what is in the field as well; it can be embedded within the tissues of the body. Emotional intelligence reveals various processes of how emotion affects our bodies and our lives. What we hold onto emotionally gets habitualized, and ritualized patterns surface. In my book, I speak about 'our inner graffiti,' the emotional writing on the wall of our cellular imprint, and what can be intuitively witnessed in the electromagnetic field. Emotional intelligence can display a wide variety of emotional states, from intense weeping to exuberant joy to deep inner peace. The emotional component is always present. But in my experience, there's never a sole cause of cancer; it's an amalgam of components."

I asked her about my friend Carol, who exercised regularly, never smoked, ate well, and still got breast cancer. Laura replied, "In situations like your friend's, there's often an emotional component. There could have been an impact that occurred long ago. It can be something as subtle as a mother leaving the room, and her child panics because she feels abandoned and doesn't have the cognitive ability to know what's going on. The child stores this in the subconscious mind, and the emotional impact affects the chemistry, the neuropatterning, and the cells of the body. Perhaps then, throughout her life, anything that has that experiential fragrance, so to speak, of being abandoned or let down will feed that energetic, chemical impact.

"Later in life, she may have had hard choices to make, like all of us do. She may have chosen to put her dreams aside. The fragrance of being abandoned eventually builds up over time and cascades into the nervous system, and the chemistry is affected to some degree. Perhaps then the endocrine system becomes more strained, and then the immune system.

"That's a very linear look at something that happens quite holographically. Again, there are many components that cause cancer, and emotional components and the resulting biochemical influence can certainly be a source. Stress, as we know, is a powerful part in the creation of disease and the breakdown of the immune system.

"It's not always like that, though. Everyone's situation is unique. In addition, there is a spiritual level of intelligence that can be a component of a condition that is ever present. It could simply be a lesson that the soul has chosen to experience.

"Many people have a serious problem with the idea that the soul is driving a condition, situation, or disease. Naturally, one would say, 'I would never have chosen this!' But that's when people lose perspective and think that this life is all there is. If one believes that the soul is an eternal consciousness, this life would then be one of many generated from their soul. Any condition is then a condition of the soul's growth, in addition to one of their current personality. The people closest to them also grow through the situation. In my view, that is what we are here to do: to grow spiritually and help others to do the same—one way or another.

"Cancer is a disease exacerbated by the lifestyles of Western culture. Toxic thoughts and stress are a huge part of this disease—just as petrochemicals and nonnutritious food are."

I asked Laura if cancer is a breakdown of the immune system, regardless of how it comes about. And she said decisively, "Yes! From a biological point of view, it's about the immune system breaking down."

Then I asked her why mainstream medical treatments use methods that compromise the immune system rather than build it up in order to help resolve the cancer cells.

"The energy around cancer is one of the most powerful structures of consciousness in our world. It's embroiled in one of the richest economic systems, right next to oil," she said.

The treatments employed by alternative centers that effectively build up the immune system rely largely on food and other natural substances—none of which can be patented, and thus, none of which can deliver the huge profits required to sustain the pharmaceutical industry.

Laura went on to say that financial gain isn't the only component that emanates from the energetic field of cancer. There is a forceful emotional thrust as well. Anyone who has had cancer knows oh so well the intense emotional turmoil that haunts them. At times, it can feel like the emotional self has been kidnapped by an evil, invisible enemy.

Laura explains it this way: "There are a lot of people who are very afraid of cancer—understandably. But the fear, and even the positive focus on research and 'running for the cure,' exists in the morphic field of cancer. The good, the bad, and death are there. The miracles, compassion, and passion to cure the disease; the lessons learned by those who have walked the path; and yes, economic greed, are all present. It's all in the field when someone utters the word or thinks the thought: 'cancer.'

"All the thoughts about cancer sustain the energy of cancer. It's a delicate balance. For example, support groups can be helpful initially, but if you keep going to them after you're cured, your system keeps being reminded of the neurological pathways that were operating when you had it. In other words, if something happens and you become afraid of snakes, then every time you think of snakes, you'll experience fear on some level. It's the same with cancer. If you're around the culture of it, you'll probably be impacted by that fearful energy, which, in the end, sustains the force behind cancer itself.

"Ridding yourself of the fear of cancer is a process, and that process is unique for everyone. Again, you have to say hello to the fear and know that it's just one energetic aspect surrounding you at any given time. At the very same time, courage, hope, love, support, and humor are within your grasp at every moment. These are equally as strong and available to you. There are always options for how you feel; it's a matter of where you put your mind's attention and focus. When you change your focus from fear to trust, for example, you change your vibration. When you change your vibration, you change the rate of the electrons and oscillations in your field. You change the imprinting and create a new set of neural pathways in your body. You change your body's chemistry in a good way. For instance, we know that laughter is good medicine and an important part of healing.

"But I can't overemphasize that whatever you focus on is what will be created. I have a client who was diagnosed with cancer in the liver and brain. She was given palliative treatment and six months to live, if that. She came to see me, and we acknowledged her doctor's diagnosis. She followed the doctor's protocols of care.

"What she also did, however, was not believe in dying. She believed in living. We intuitively created affirming, healing slogans for her situation that truly matched her emotional and spiritual intelligence and created a healing inner environment for her body chemistry and organs. She wrote them down on paper and taped them all around her house. She had some touch-and-go moments, but five years later, she is currently hiking with her dogs up the mountains by her home and visiting the oceans of California, both of which are healing to her. She knows—*believes*—that she is well. The doctors call her their miracle patient."

Once again Laura reiterated a message that runs throughout this book: it's vital to your healing process to position yourself in a place of positive thoughts, and to focus on what you want rather than what you don't want. "One of the biggest agents for healing is a happiness that reflects a deeper level of contentment. Being at peace changes your electromagnetic field, as does being angry or afraid. It changes the field around your body and the electromagnetic fields around your cells. Cells talk to each other, and the electromagnetic fields flare or spike when emotions are prevalent. In my experience, as I witness spikes of emotion that are fearful, the energy around my cells becomes thicker and less responsive, and so do the cells themselves over time.

"Conversely, when there is peace and happiness, you create a body of happiness. There is emotional softness, feelings of safety and relaxation. When you can organically say, 'I love my life,' you'll know you're there.

"To truly know the healing power within, you have to recognize the eternal nature of who you are. The more you get that, the more you have access to your infinite power. The clearer and more stable the connection to your infinite power, the more in touch you are with what *is* and, therefore, what you need in this moment to heal, to be healthy, and to live fully."

I asked Laura to elaborate on infinite power in relation to what some would call miraculous healing or spontaneous remission, but what I have come to believe is quite common.

"Infinite power is there whether there is a spontaneous miracle involved or not." She affirmed, "For those who experience spontaneous remission, that is simply their life path—it's what's supposed to happen for them. When I look at their energy, I see that they had the connection to the power needed to make that happen as part of their life path. Not everyone has spontaneous remission in their destiny, but if you don't connect, you won't know. And if you do connect, you'll find peace—genuine peace—no matter the outcome.

"Spontaneous remissions happen quickly. In a simplistic view, you could look at it this way. We are energy, or frozen light, and when healing occurs, the pattern of light rebalances quickly, moving away from an incongruence or disease. We are, after all, a field of quantum soup.

"It's a delicate process to discuss spontaneous healings in such a short time. With that being said, it won't happen for someone if it's not supposed to happen. One of the many insights I learned from my own near-death experience is that no matter what is going on in your life, if you were supposed to be somewhere else, you would be."

This led us into a discussion of destiny. Is destiny the only way you can experience such healing, or is there some measure of choice? Laura replied, "When you connect to the power of who you are—God or Source—you understand that you have choices in some aspects of life's experience. In other aspects, you simply get to experience them. That has been my observation in my own life and the lives of my clients. You can choose to heal. When you connect with Source, you may realize that it's not your time to heal, that perhaps there is another plan. This is a hard concept for people to get behind, because no one wants to be sick, let alone die. This is not about giving up on yourself. It's about being real with *this* moment. Being in the moment and connected is where miracles exist, not in wishful thinking.

"I am a firm believer in both destiny and free will because both are true. There is destiny, and there is free will and willpower. Free will is about choice. When you use your intuition with free will to make a choice—including the choice to heal from cancer—you usually make the choices that are correct for your path and not based on your lower egoic nature. If you make a choice that goes against your path, you'll get a lot of interesting lessons along the way, but eventually your intuitive voice will turn you toward the balanced point and acceptance. Acceptance is not giving up. The feeling of 'giving up' is egoic and never lasts for very long.

"Willpower is the determined thoughts and subsequent energy you use in order to support both the choice of free will and the choice derived from intuitive knowing. Often people use willpower to beat themselves up. Others claim that they just don't have the will to do something. I say, 'Yes, you do.' Use that will to keep yourself from quitting.

"Keep this in mind: it takes a tremendous amount of willpower to stay unhealthy or poor. Conditions such as these result from not listening to what you know *is* true for you.

"Life in a body is all about evolution. You may have come in with the predisposition for cancer as an experience, but if you learn the lessons from it, you have a high probability of shifting that paradigm. It's true in all areas of life. Like if you've been dating the same kind of guy forever and keep having bad experiences, and then suddenly you meet someone who rocks your world. You have to use your intuition to know if this is going to be the same book, with a slightly different cover, or if this person is really different because you yourself have changed deep inside.

"By using your intuition, you can stand on the edge of a forthcoming experience and sense its nature. You can intuitively assess the inherent lessons and perhaps choose to go through the experience again, or you can let it go. If you let it go before entering into it, you can check that series of lessons off your list. When you do, you can heal.

"The same is true with cancer. The best way out of cancer is to follow the voice of your soul and use everything God put on this earth to help you heal. And as I said, the biggest component of that healing is how you position your thoughts so that you can vibrate in alignment with healing and deep inner contentment."

Laura went on to explain that all of life's challenges, including cancer, can be an opening door. "Disease, chaos, or problems are all opportunities to recognize your eternal nature and your inherent connective power to make changes. They are ways to both verify and fortify you through the use of your intuition. Intuition, your inner wisdom, is the vehicle that allows you access to the infinite nature of who you are. Logic won't take you there, but it will help you put intuitive answers into perspective and to create a strategy. Emotions won't help you get there; intuition is the way. Intuition is your soul speaking with you about *you.*"

I think some people may fear relying on intuition because of what others might think. Laura provided good medicine: "There's always going to be someone who doesn't believe what you believe. The love you have for yourself is not predicated on someone else's approval. The mission you have here on this earth is the gift."

Still, many people believe that when something "bad" happens, it's because of karma or past-life issues. Laura agrees that karma could be part of the mix. "Past lives can have an influence, but I like people to take a broader perspective, because past lives are not relevant. So what if you were raped in Bulgaria or trampled by a mastodon? So what? Our soul has done so many things; it has myriad experiences. It's almost futile to try and tie them all together around this one experience. Every death experience follows you and has lessons embedded within it. Everything is a hash mark, a notch on your soul's wall. When you learn from it, you can check it off.

"Then again, if you *feel* that looking into past-life information is important, use your intuition to learn from it."

Laura's closing message was a bright reminder about keeping perspective. "Keep in mind that even though it's more intense here because you're in a body with a nervous system driving sensations and experiences into your life, we do more work on the other side than we do here. One of my favorite sayings is, 'Life is a working vacation for your soul.' When you're here on earth, you tend to forget that you are eternal light. I know the day-to-day can be traumatic when you're struggling with a diagnosis. I have been there; trust me, I know. However, the power of your inner wakefulness and your ability to bring that power into the moment is influential medicine. Love your body and your amazing personality. Then, first and foremost, honor, connect with, and love your soul. That is where healing happens."

To learn more about Laura Alden Kamm, go to energymedicine.org.

The golden opportunity you are seeking is in yourself. It is not in your environment, it is not in luck or chance or the hope of others; it is in yourself alone.
ORISON SWETT MARDEN

KENT TOMPKINS, LPC, CCH

Spiritual Healing

Life begets life. Energy creates energy. It is by spending oneself that one becomes rich.
SARAH BERNHARDT

I met Kent Tompkins serendipitously. I was planning a surprise party for my mother's eightieth birthday, but was disgruntled at the prices that resorts wanted for party rooms, lodging, and food. I figured the best way around the expense was by landing a private home where my family could sleep, where we could have the party, and where a caterer could bring the food. Oh, and a nice view would work, too.

Looking skyward, I said, "OK, God. I need that house. Thank you."

The very next day I received an e-mail from Kent. He belongs to the same online network as I do, and Kent was letting the group know that he was making his house available for yoga retreats, workshops, family reunions, and so on. My grin filled the room. I read further: not only was the price reasonable, but the location of the house was also in my mother's favorite spot in Colorado.

It was a no-brainer. "Thank you, God," I said again, smiling gratefully.

Weeks later, I drove to the house to check it out. Kent and I began to talk beyond the logistics of where to set up tables and the best spot for the buffet line. I learned that he was a licensed professional counselor and hypnotherapist. He'd also lived on Navajo and White Mountain Apache lands for many years and studied ceremonial healing with elders in the Navajo and Southern Cheyenne Indian tribes, all the while documenting sacred sites through a camera lens. I learned these things as he walked me down a path to a space he had cleared for a tepee, where he would eventually perform ceremonial rituals.

I told Kent about this book. He nodded and looked deeply into my eyes. "My mother died of cancer in 1977. I decided that if I really wanted to learn about healing, I had to learn how to heal cancer."

Our conversation took off from there. A few weeks later, I conducted a formal interview with him.

***

"Ever since I was a child," Tompkins began, "I saw energy and could sense things. There wasn't any reinforcement about how to work with that, but there was a voice inside me that I trusted. I was especially grounded whenever I was out in nature, so I was in nature every chance I got.

"It wasn't until I stepped foot on the Navajo reservation and was invited into ceremonies that things began to gel for me. That's when I understood the context of what I had perceived as a child."

When Tompkins's mother was diagnosed with cancer, he had not yet learned the way of the Navajo. But he did help his mother work with a doctor out of California named Carl Simonton (Simonton Cancer Center, simontoncen ter.com).

"Dr. Simonton is a cutting-edge guy who came up with cancer personality types. My mother fit it to the letter. Before she got colon cancer, she was filled with helplessness and hopelessness. She was also very heavy. I journeyed with her for eighteen months before she died, but through working with Dr. Simonton, she learned a lot about why the cancer had shown up. So did I. In the end, she took full ownership of choosing cancer and found ways to abate it for a period of time."

According to Tompkins, cancer can result from thought forms that an individual adopts at a very early age. These thought forms get compartmentalized in the body and block specific energetic pathways. He explained it further: "Everything in the universe is created from the same Divine spark, including humans.

Everything operates at a certain frequency. Atoms vibrate at a certain frequency, and various parts of the atom vibrate at different frequencies. Each human being has a different vibration and frequency, which is based on what they hold in their thoughts. Thought forms direct energy. So for example, if the person holds a great deal of shame or guilt, those thought forms will stifle the flow of energy.

"Conversely, imagine love as an integrating force, which it is. Imagine love as that moment in time or that state of being in which harmony, beauty, and divine intelligence merge. In this living, breathing state of being, energy flows unencumbered throughout our physical, emotional, mental, and spiritual bodies. These conditions activate the parasympathetic nervous system, which then boosts the immune system. Then endorphins kick in, and the body's natural morphine elevates mood, heals, and restores wellness.

"In this state of being, we have enhanced intuitive abilities, and the fight-or-flight response is diminished. Consequently, there's a greater potential for continually creating an atmosphere of self-healing, both physical and emotional.

"When we allow ourselves to be intuitively led to that which is right for us, right now, then one moment is always morphing into the next—right now. We lose our concept of linear time and the attachment to specific outcomes that our egos perceive as significant. This signals that we are entering a state of continual healing and wellness. Living a whole and spiritual life is one that's unpredictable to the ego and often confusing to the brain. Yet in this place of intuitive awareness, we are connected to the true nature of our souls."

If this sounds like an ambitious adventure and one that requires a map or some other form of guidance, it is. Still, every journey starts with the first step, and Tompkins believes the journey of self-healing begins by addressing negative thought forms. "My work is to assist clients in recognizing thought forms that aren't serving them. Maybe they got them from their parents, from religion, from teachers. It doesn't matter. What matters is that they start to see negative thought patterns that they took for granted, not realizing that these thoughts created adverse energy shifts in their bodies, minds, and souls.

"Once they see the thoughts, they can unravel them and create new ones that are more in line with who they really are. When that happens, people almost immediately feel an energy shift in their bodies and minds. That creates a different frequency that delivers energy into those areas that were closed off before. In this manner, clients are shifting energy within themselves, applying various laws of physics, and becoming more accountable for their wellness. Healing cancer has to do with opening up energy flows into the areas that were once closed off."

Tompkins says shame commonly blocks energy flow. "When a parent reprimands a small child for doing what's natural for small children, the child tends to focus on believing something is wrong with him rather than returning to that intuitive state of natural curiosity, learning, and love. When a child is repeatedly told, either verbally or nonverbally, that his behavior is wrong, the potential is set for his acceptance of the negative thought forms, and then he possibly begins to believe to a varying degree that it's not OK to be who he really is. That's when 'simply being' is replaced with shame or guilt.

"This belief system sifts down to the subconscious mind, and very often the child attempts to heal the parent, significant other, or the family dynamic that delivered the disintegrated message, rather than heal the self. Eventually, the subconscious beliefs, to a marked degree, determine the individual's way of life and can manifest as disease.

"Disease can be viewed as self-sabotaging behavior, the decrease of natural curiosity, or any negative thought form that deconstructs the human's natural constitution of wellness. And when there's more disintegration than integration, when the stressors tax the body and mind, things get very unbalanced. There are so many more stressors now than ever before. Frequencies get skewed; energy gets blocked. That's one way to look at how cancer comes about. But it's a big topic."

That topic is so big, in fact, that when I asked Tompkins about why some people get cancer and others don't—even though we're all exposed to a barrage of stressors—he admitted that it's a mystery. "The obvious answer is that those who are most out of balance are most susceptible. But research doesn't warrant that. Then you throw in environmental toxins, the changes in the quality of the food we eat, radio waves, and all the electronic gadgets—there are so many variables. I am still gaining the wisdom to understand the bigger picture.

"If we could have the insight into each person's soul to see what their design really is, why the person came here at this time and chose to experience life this way, it would reveal so much. That's what I'm most curious about. I believe if we could experience a *knowing* of ourselves rather than spending time fighting against something; if we could embrace all aspects of ourselves, whether it's cancer or a torn meniscus; if we could really and truly arrive at *knowing* what's behind the cancer, then we could stop all the subconscious negative influences and see the soul's story. That's when the core truth is revealed."

Tompkins brought the conversation back to what he believes is at the heart of what heals. "Love, as the integrating force, is like a liquid nectar, a honey that gets crystallized when these disintegrating messages are dominant. In truth, love is all there is. Everything else is misdirected energy. So you can see how valuable it is to empower self-discovery and to honor childhood innocence, not only in children, but also within each other and within our communities.

"When I work with people, I observe them gaining awareness about where those pockets of energy are blocked. When they change the frequency, then the crystallized structure turns back into nectar, and they are back on the road to living in their power. Intuitive energy flows again. They understand themselves as spiritual beings without having to pay homage to misguided thought forms any longer."

Accessing the healing power of love and that *knowing* he speaks of starts simply with a desire to be more aware. Becoming truly aware entails diligence and discipline that we may not have previously employed. "By the time cancer strikes the body," Tompkins said, "there's probably been five years of warning signs that have presented themselves to the individual. They may be subtle at first, like a faint wisp of wind saying, 'You're hanging with the wrong people' or 'You'd better get into the right work.'

"Life is all about self-discovery, which requires awareness, yet we can ease into it slowly. We can start to notice if we're living our right timing, doing the right work, engaging in the right relationships, and honoring our intuition. When we aren't doing those things, we aren't in our power. We're giving it away. Illness is a symbol from the body, and that symbol is trying to wake us up. It gets louder and louder, until eventually we get sick. Cancer is one of the loudest symbols; it's our body screaming at us to live with more integrity and accountability.

"In our culture, tending to ourselves when we're healthy and well is not as customary as it is within the Chinese, Native American, or East Indian cultures. Our culture, as a rule, does not celebrate and pray that wellness continues, nor does it reinforce what's going right. Instead we ignore the warning signs as long as we can. We wait until we're sick before we pay attention. We have a hard time changing until we get cut off at the knees."

The good news is that even after ignoring the signs for years on end, we can still heal, either with the help of others or by accessing the God-given power within. "People can absolutely heal themselves," Tompkins affirmed. "It happens all the time. But how many people actually think it's possible? It takes enormous courage and integrity to live within the mystery, without seemingly clear answers or direction. Yet it is precisely within this mystery that surrender to spirit occurs and our higher selves bond with the nourishment and guidance we need. To the brain, this process is very foreign.

"Believing in yourself is the first step," he continued, "and so is accepting your right to live as a free agent. Understand that you are obligated to no one. Say yes when you mean yes and no when you mean no. Give of yourself and be of service, absolutely, but create a balance of honesty about where to place your allegiance. Live and share out of joy, not fear.

"Visit your own intuition. Sit with it. Get a quieter mind. It takes practice, but intuition will never let you down. Your brain will try to pull you away, but once you arrive at a *knowing* of something and eventually know who you really are, you'll be OK.

"Ask yourself, 'Who do I work for? Who's my boss?' You need to find the divine link with something—not necessarily another human being, although teachers are great. But good teachers always tell you to question everything they say; they test you and say you have to find it within yourself."

There are models and teachers out there, Tompkins told me, but we typically find them in unorthodox ways.

That alone can lend to inner doubt and outer criticism. Tompkins then told me the story of one of his best teachers, a Navajo elder. "I knocked on his door every day for at least a year, wanting to work with him. Instead, he'd tell me to move a pile of dirt from one place in his yard to another, or to load up the kids and take them somewhere. I moved tires from here to there, and took building supplies up to his summer camp above Black Mesa, deep in the Navajo rez. He had me do chores for an entire year.

"There were times when I wanted to quit, but my Navajo friends urged me to stick with it. Finally, he knocked on my door late one night and said, 'Are you ready?' and I said, 'Yes.'

"This is a guy who died in battle in the Korean War, had had an out-of-body experience, woke up in the hospital, and became a healer from that day forward. For six years, night and day, every day of the week, I witnessed him do healings that Westerners would call miracles—difficult cases that would require an operating room for most doctors. But he used a buffalo horn, a pocketknife, fire, and water. He never turned anyone away. He told me that to truly be of service and allow the One Creator to flow through, he had to put all judgment aside. In essence, the one that knows nothing knows everything! He never charged money, only asked for donations. He and his wife went on to adopt twelve kids."

For reasons we may never understand, Tompkins's teacher and eventual colleague was able to access and practice the art of healing after his near-death experience. But Tompkins says we don't have to go to that extreme to tap into our own source of healing. It does help, though, to find a mentor who can assist with the process—and it *is* a process. "Get off the beaten track and believe that you amount to something. Then look for a good, open-minded, spiritually oriented therapist, counselor, guide, or teacher. Trust your intuition. Seek a like-minded person. Study how they live, how they go about things. Teachers can be hard to find, so you need to set a strong intention. Affirm to yourself that you are in the process of finding the right healer. Affirm that you are walking down the path, and it is unfolding.

"When you find a possible mentor, ask for fifteen minutes of their time. If after that it doesn't feel right, ask for three referrals and leave. Keep moving. It's like a treasure hunt. You might get a sign after looking under the first rock, but you might turn over twelve rocks and find nothing. Doesn't matter. Keep moving. It's all about being dedicated to the treasure hunt.

"We're going to see a quickening of all these things. We're demystifying ideas about how difficult it is to heal oneself. More people are using spiritual approaches to healing. These people are recognizing the power of themselves as an integrated whole. They are experiencing how shifting one's thought forms has a direct impact on how the body responds. My clients are able to arrive at knowing that there are no limits, except those that they impose on themselves or those that they have yet to uncover. It leaves little room for denial, blaming of others, and the lure of falling asleep spiritually.

"Some people give up because they feel foolish or defeated. But I know that if there is a desire in your heart to be well, there will be a teacher or healer for you. Desires don't exist deeply in your heart unless the answer and ultimate manifestation of those desires also exist. So step up. Have courage. And dedicate yourself to wellness."

Tompkins's conviction is reinforced by his belief that we are supported in ways beyond our normal understanding. "Humans are gifted with free will. With that, we make choices about whether or not to seek help when our bodies give us signals that things aren't right—or to deny the help we're given. We have free will to be closed to the mystery of life or to be open and learn something new. We are granted the opportunity to wake up and grow over and over again.

"You can ask for help from the invisible, and your journey can then kick into turbo gear. But you have to be open to receive the gifts. If you put your hand out and ask for help, then you are signifying that you are receptive to change. If your hand is closed, however, no one has the right to pry it open and insist that you take what they have to offer. What is your intention? How ready are you to open your hand and risk changing?

"The invisible assistants are here to help. Jesus is one of my bosses, and I enjoy a wonderful relationship with St. Francis. But neither would think of interfering with my free will. Yet they will be there in a nanosecond with unlimited grace if they see that I am running myself into a ditch. These nonphysical assistants and teachers honor us so much that they allow us to go to cancerous stages. They simply won't interfere. The level of respect they maintain for the free will that humans have in this school called life is unwavering. Still, they're waiting for us to ask for help, and when we do—with an open hand and heart—it comes pouring in.

"We are never alone. We have been led; we are being led; and we will be led."

As inspiring as that is, Tompkins also acknowledged that the mix of free will, intention, negative thought forms, cultural shortsightedness, and the loving assistance from the nonphysical calls up as much mystery as it does possibility. "If we can surrender to the mystery, release our attachment to outcomes, and, hence, arrive at *knowing* ourselves and the Creator, then we're on the path," he said with marvel in his voice. "Humans are inherently complete, yet due to blind spots, we perceive ourselves as incomplete. So we're constantly trying to bring ourselves back into balance. That's how we grow.

"Be patient, keep searching, keep moving. After you begin to realize the power that flows through you, be humble. Accepting one's power with humility and maintaining this presence is the goal. The healing power is the divine spark flowing through you. Let it vibrate in every cell in your body and say, 'Thank you.'"

To learn more about Kent Tompkins and his work, go to invisionwellness.com or kentart.com.

I get up. I walk.
I fall down.
Meanwhile, I keep dancing.
RABBI HILLEL

CHAPTER 9

Fortitude

*Courage is the human virtue that counts
most—courage to act on limited
knowledge and insufficient evidence.
That's all any of us have.*
ROBERT FROST

Each day, we're challenged to do what's necessary to heal. We select the path that's right for us. Maybe it's chemo and radiation. Maybe it's herbs and supplements. Maybe meditation and visualization. Or it could be a combination of those things. What we choose is less relevant than our *belief* in what we're doing and our commitment to it.

The greatest challenge of getting from here to there is in the mind. We are well conditioned when it comes to cancer. Nobody ever looked at me with delight and said, "Oh, what a wonderful opportunity to evolve into your next stage of life!" Rather, a diagnosis is fraught with grotesque images and terrifying statistics. People respond gravely to the very word. Because of their conditioning, many people carry the fear that you and everyone else with cancer will die. We even think and feel those things ourselves, which is in no way helpful.

To allow the deepest level of healing to occur, and certainly to support ourselves fully, it's critically important to patrol the thoughts that enter our mind. This is the den where whatever enters and stays will expand. So even though fear, doubt, sorrow, anger, and many other emotionally laden thoughts will come knocking, it's up to us to manage what stays and what goes.

It's fruitless to pretend that these heavy emotions don't exist. They're a normal crowd that parades through the complex experience of a cancer diagnosis. Still, if healing is what you're after, then it's wise to entertain the negative band of thoughts for a time and then boot them out like a cadre of drunks who have crashed the party. Invite healing thoughts to stay in their place. Build them a room in the house of your mind. Make them very comfortable. Listen to them often.

I continue to retrain myself out of my addiction to drama and negative thinking by reading books and listening to CDs about the value of focusing on forgiveness, beauty, gratitude, compassion, patience, and the other attributes of love. We're fortunate to be living in a time where there are hundreds—maybe thousands—of books that can cleanse us of our ill-fated mental and emotional habits. It sounds too simple to pack such a miraculous punch, but by letting go of those oppressive cognitive coots, we can heal very deeply and profoundly.

Of course, letting go of oppressive thoughts and healing deeply are easier said than done. We live in a culture of black-and-white answers, right and wrong people, them against us, my loss due to their fault. To defrock this way of thinking, we have to want and trust our own authority. We have to want to transcend a societal mandate that finds fault in others while taking care not to reveal our own vulnerabilities and culpabilities. It takes courage, in the most mythic sense of the word, to break the habit of finding others guilty of our misery and downfall, and to assume full responsibility for our lives.

When we do this, however, liberation becomes the dance partner in life and freedom becomes the reward. It's a beautiful thing to know that you and your divine inner self are in charge of the party. That's when the gripes and screams of others are barely audible, because all you notice, all you focus on, is the infinite good that exists both within yourself and lining every cloud in the sky.

It takes practice to stop scrutinizing the other person or circumstance and making them the scapegoat. When you're on the path to true healing, every conflict comes back to you and how you are responding to the emotions within the dynamic. You can no longer point to what's "out there" as the problem, which means it's not about your doctor, your parents, your spouse, your children, your job, or your cancer, and how you feel wronged by those things. It's about *you* and how you are going to be with *you* around those feelings so you can be free.

It's sometimes unnerving to have to suck it up and relinquish blame. It's just so much easier to point fingers! Healing from the pollution of finding fault continues to be a lifelong ambition. That it takes fortitude is an understatement, but acquiescing to spiritual evolution and knowing what love is *really* about is the very source of the glimmer in our eyes and the rhythm in our step. There's nothing sweeter than that.

Your life becomes the thing you have decided it shall be.

RAYMOND CHARLES BARKER

DIANE'S STORY

If you treat an individual as if he were what he ought to be and could be, he will become what he ought to be and could be.
JOHANN WOLFGANG VON GOETHE

After three cancer diagnoses, Diane became a cancer coach and began to help others grasp the underlying emotional energy that may have contributed to the disease. However, not until her fourth diagnosis did she begin asking herself the same questions that she posed to her clients, questions that she herself had been avoiding because they were too painful to address personally.

Like most people in this book, Diane thinks emotional components are important and significant reasons why people get the disease. Her cancer journey has been a long one, but her courage is steadfast. She continues to uproot self-sabotaging beliefs that she perceives are detrimental to her well-being.

Diane's harrowing story is, at first, a typical scenario, but then emerges into a beautiful and unique tale of self-discovery. It all began in 1995 when a golf-ball-sized lump suddenly appeared under her left armpit. Her doctor thought it was just a fatty tumor. A few months later, egged on by a gut feeling, she visited a breast cancer specialist. The specialist also proclaimed that it was nothing, and a needle biopsy validated the good news. Even so, Diane wanted the lump removed.

Six months after initially finding the lump, and two benign biopsies later, she had surgery. The results were not good. As her surgeon explained, "You have at least two lumps, and they could be many different things. Have you ever heard of Hodgkin's disease?"

Indeed she had. A family friend had died from it. Diane was in shock as she underwent a battery of tests. "When I told my mom, she began sobbing. Her brother had been diagnosed with terminal lung cancer that very same day. On top of that, when I was nine months old, she had lost a son, my little brother. The idea of losing another child must have been overwhelming. At that moment, I went into crisis-management mode for everyone else. I felt like I had to be strong for them." And so began Diane's turn on what she calls the "cancer conveyor belt."

Diane had stage 1 lymphocyte-predominant Hodgkin's disease with twelve cancerous lymph nodes. The doctor told her it was in the earliest stage and easily curable. After she knew the whole story, she visited a naturopathic doctor that her pastor had recommended. "The ND told me not to do chemo and that he could heal me with high doses of vitamin C. I thought he was crazy, and so I went ahead with the chemo and radiation. But he did talk me into taking a powdered form of vitamin C and a vitamin E supplement to help my skin during radiation."

Diane underwent eight months of chemo and two months of radiation. She also worked two jobs during her treatment and took two night classes to avoid facing the situation. "If I stopped moving, even for a second, I was afraid I'd cry. More importantly, I was afraid I'd never stop crying.

"I was exhausted. I'd get the chemo, go home, and be sick all weekend. I was in a lot of pain, and I was very concerned about my mom seeing me in pain. I had insomnia because of it. My nerves were on fire, and the weight of my own body was excruciating. At night, my mom would come in and say good night, and as soon as she'd leave, I'd get out of bed and sit on the floor and rock back and forth, back and forth, until I collapsed from exhaustion. The pain was unbearable."

The radiation wasn't as difficult—until she ran out of the vitamin E. After only a few days of not taking it, she developed third-degree burns in her underarms.

Those of us who enter the world of cancer are trained to accept the idea that chemo and radiation are harsh, but if they work, it's worth the pain and suffering. We understand that people sacrifice comfort (both in the short and long term) so they can then resume and live out a long healthy life. That's the idea, anyhow.

It seemed to have worked for Diane. She passed the five-year survival mark and became one of the statistics that cite a victory, a *cure,* from using the standard fare. What those statistics on't take into account, however, is what happens after five years. That's when conventional medicine stops keeping track.

One year after she was pronounced cancer free and six years after her first diagnosis, Diane's cancer came back "with a vengeance." This time it was located in lymph nodes throughout her body. This time it was stage 3. This time the same cancer she had before was now called "incurable."

So much for sacrificing comfort for a long, healthy life.

"I had already decided that if the cancer ever came back, I wouldn't do chemo and radiation again. But of course, that's all the doctors had to offer. I was told to go see a specialist about a bone-marrow transplant. I said, 'If this is incurable, why would I put myself through that?' It didn't make any sense."

The next few weeks were a blur. Diane brazenly announced to her family that she was refusing treatment. She went on a vacation with friends, but it was interrupted by the shocking events on 9/11. "I tried to process what had happened. It occurred to me that every person who died in that tragedy had no choice. Something shifted inside me. I thought, 'I have a choice. How dare I choose to die? There's got to be a way to heal in a more humane way, a way that resonates with me and my beliefs.'"

She conducted an in-depth Internet search, during which Daniel Rubin, an Arizona-based naturopath, came up several times. While reviewing his website, Diane noticed that he used vitamin C to upregulate the immune system so the body can fight off the cancer on its own. According to Diane, "Bells and whistles went off. I thought, 'Yeah, it's in my immune system, in my lymphatic system. Why wouldn't that work?'"

Within days, she was in Scottsdale talking to Dr. Rubin.

"When I walked in, I felt a difference in the atmosphere immediately. First and foremost, it felt and looked alive; never before had a treatment room felt like that. After a routine workup, I sat down with Dr. Rubin. After twenty-five minutes of questions about my life, such as 'What do you do?' and 'Tell us about your support network' and 'Have your parents passed away? If so, how?' I thought 'Wait, I'm paying you good money, and you're not even asking about my cancer?'

"And then, out of the blue, Dr. Rubin asked who the woodworker was in my family. I was stunned. My father had been a woodworker. Dr. Rubin then asked, 'Did he use treated lumber? Were you exposed to it? Did you know that treated lumber has copper in it and lymphocyte-predominant Hodgkin's is directly correlated to high copper levels?' Dr. Rubin knew more about this disease than any other doctor ever had—even though they all had access to the same medical journals."

Diane felt a strong connection and desire to work with Dr. Rubin, but decided it was prudent to get another MD's perspective as well. The doctor she saw was new to her, but within minutes of hearing her diagnosis, he was certain about the protocol: ten months of chemo and a bone-marrow transplant.

"I asked him why he wanted to be so aggressive if this disease was considered incurable. He promised me that we could kick it with this approach. I told him I didn't want to be sick for ten months, and he said, 'Honey, you have cancer. You're probably going to be a very sick young woman for the next two years.'"

Diane requested that he provide a list of all the drugs they would use, along with a description of both the short- and long-term side effects. The doctor agreed and also said he would make sure that Rituxin, his choice of chemo, would work with her type of cancer.

When she returned a few weeks later, the doctor neglected to provide a list of side effects, nor had he determined if Rituxin would be appropriate. Diane handed him Dr. Rubin's file and asked for feedback on the protocol. The doctor flipped through the pages and told her it was "a bunch of crap" and "none of that stuff works." After over an hour of heated discussion and debate, Diane was stunned when he said, "Go on your three-week vacation to Scottsdale, and when you come back, we'll have to start all over."

She retorted that it was a twelve-week minimum protocol, to which he declared adamantly, "You'll be dead in twelve weeks."

With financial help from family and friends, Diane was soon in Arizona. This is where the real story of her healing begins. "I received supplements and vitamin C IVs, and I did a variety of complementary therapies, such as colon hydrotherapy, lymphatic-drainage massage, and oxygen-ozone saunas. However, the lifestyle changes and emotional journey were what created the real healing. Living in a hotel room by myself, 2,400 miles away from home, I had time to go within myself and work on the emotional wounds that had brought me to that life-changing moment."

Diane pursued exercises to cleanse her mind, spirit, and body. It wasn't easy. She changed her eating habits and thought processes, developed self-empowerment and stress-management techniques, and began journaling.

Then one day at the clinic, a woman asked Diane if she loved herself. "I remember laughing in my head. I replied with 'Of course I do,' a hint of sarcasm oozing from me. She asked again, 'No, do you really love yourself? When you look in the mirror and say "I love you," do you feel it in your cells?' I got up with my IV pole and excused myself to the bathroom. When I returned, I put on my headset and went to sleep."

Yet when Diane woke the next morning, the question was still lingering. She looked into the mirror, laughed, and said, "I love you," but she felt nothing. She repeated it again and again. Nothing. "I started to cry. I realized that not only did I not love myself, but I didn't even know how."

She canceled treatment that day and sat in front of the mirror for hours, reading every card and letter that people had sent to her, until she finally began to believe in her value. "A crack in my consciousness occurred, and I saw that I was worthy of love and I did love myself as a child of God—unconditionally. After that, everything seemed to click."

Diane had always projected a positive and upbeat personality, but now it shone even brighter. And people noticed. After her treatments were complete, she left Arizona and returned to her home in New York. She was happy.

Two years later, she was hit with her third diagnosis. It was the same type of cancer as the first two diagnoses. This time, she followed a more traditional protocol by enduring four rounds of Rituxin. But after experiencing several bouts of rare side effects, Diane left her support system in New York and moved to Arizona.

With the cancer once again in remission, things went well. She married, landed a great job, and made friends. She took classes to become a life coach so she could help others going through their life transitions, including cancer. She hired Richard, a spiritual life coach, to coach her. Their work together was highly effective and stirred up things that surprised her.

"During one of our sessions, it became clear that deep inside me, I was incredibly pissed off that the cancer had come back a third time. I was able to work through those emotions in the next two sessions, just in time to be diagnosed a fourth time.

"From 2008 to the beginning of 2010, I went for naturopathic treatments, reclaimed my good eating habits, and did all of the external things I needed to do. But I avoided looking at my deeper emotional self at all costs. It was a contradiction, though, because as a life coach that's exactly where I take my clients. I knew the answers were within, but I just didn't want to go any deeper than I already had."

During those two years, Diane's scans came back looking better in some places, worse in others, but consistently showing slow growth of the existing tumors. After two solid years of what Diane refers to as "hide-and-seek cancer," she decided it was time to roll up her sleeves, put on her life-coach cap, and ask herself the tough questions. In the process, she identified every extreme emotional upset that had occurred within two years prior to each of her diagnoses.

The inquiry led to a veritable jackpot. Before every new diagnosis, a life-draining event had impacted her.

They included the death of her father and mother, severe financial hardships, and finally, a festering anger that brewed after her third diagnosis and that she believes prompted the fourth.

"Lymphoma is a free-flowing cancer. Although it resides in the lymph nodes, lymphatic fluid travels, and its role is to pick up the body's toxins and remove them. But mine weren't removing the toxins. My nodes were hanging on to toxins as if for dear life. I began to think on this." Diane wrote down the following questions:

- What is the cancer and/or toxin that is flowing throughout my life that I am holding on to?
- How does cancer serve me?
- The cancer is located primarily in my stomach and under my breastbone. What does this represent?

She left the questions in her journal and allowed a nonrational, subconscious process to turn the soil for an answer. Meanwhile, she began using neurofeedback, a system that uses electrodes to help access deep-seated beliefs and create healthy, balanced brainwaves (see optimumbalancing.com). In one session, Diane asked herself, "What do I need to know to heal this cancer once and for all?"

"I suddenly saw a huge umbilical cord come out from my stomach and a pair of scissors cutting it. Tons of blood oozed out, and I thought, 'Cut the cord. I just need to cut the cord.' I had just arrived at the deepest understanding of my soul's need for cancer."

As she reflected on the questions and events around her diagnoses, more pieces of her puzzle came together. In 1992, just days before her father passed away, Diane found out—by chance—that she was not his biological child. She said, "This was an incredible blow to my identity. For twenty-two years, I had believed I was the daughter of this man who epitomized integrity, values, and morals. Suddenly, I learned that he wasn't my dad, even though he loved me like an exceptional father would love his daughter. Then he died. He didn't know I knew the truth. I never got to say thank you. My heart broke that day, and my identity was buried with the man I called Dad."

That wasn't all. She also learned that her biological father had died a month before she was born and that her mother had hidden her pregnancy from everyone until days after Diane was born, telling people that the hospital visit was for stomach surgery.

"I began to think about what my mom thought of me while I was in the womb. It was 1969, and she was a single mother with four kids, divorced, dating, and now pregnant with another child. I am not sure if she planned on keeping me or giving me up, but I am certain she wasn't happy about being pregnant. Hiding her pregnancy indicates to me that she was ashamed of me. I definitely wasn't getting loving messages in the womb."

Diane elaborated on her mother's nature. "She expected perfection out of me. It was unhealthy, but I didn't realize how bad it was until later in life. My mom's love had conditions—conditions that disappeared the day I was diagnosed with cancer. Suddenly, I no longer had to be perfect; I just had to live.

"I realized important things after I delved into the lost parts of myself: First, cancer had become my new identity after I lost my father. Next, I had spent thirty-nine years of my life trying to prove that I was good enough, that I deserved to be here, and that I deserved to be loved for who I am.

"With all my heart, I know on a spiritual level that I contracted with my mom and everyone else in my life to learn this lesson of self-love. I am incredibly grateful that these "ahas" came after my mom passed so that the wonderful bond and friendship we created after our initial healing remained intact. She passed knowing that she was my best friend and that I loved her very much."

Remarkably, in the process of this awakening, Diane's menses started, and the amount of blood and clots she expelled was equivalent to a miscarriage. "Cancer was my pregnancy—the manifestation of unhealthy emotions and unlovable thoughts," she said, "but I've finally cut the cord. Since the day I was *conceived,* I had been trying to prove that I deserve to be here."

When she had that realization, she knew she had hit the source of her cancer.

Diane still works with a homeopathic doctor to help heal on the deepest levels. "I'm looking forward to my next scan. Since things have changed and healed within me on a spiritual and emotional level, I trust I will heal physically as well. I don't need the cancer anymore. It's fulfilled its role, and now I can move on. My energy is better than it's ever been, and everyone around me says how much younger and more vibrant I look.

"Richard, my spiritual life coach, says, 'Go within or go without.' I agree completely."

Diane recently had a dream that repeated the phrase "thirty-nine plus one." She interprets the dream in this way: "I spent the first thirty-nine years of my life creating situations, including cancer, to show me what my soul's lesson was. And now, at age forty (thirty-nine plus one), I'm living the first year of the rest of my life."

Diane continues coaching others about the physical manifestation of emotional and spiritual pain. "Helping others to help themselves makes being on this journey worth every bit of pain and heartache. Asking hard questions can take us on the adventure of a lifetime. It's a ride you'll never forget and never regret."

To learn more about Diane, go to d ianeparadise.com or visit naturalcancer girl.com.

The courage to be is the courage to accept oneself in spite of being unacceptable.
PAUL TILLICH

DANIEL RUBIN, ND, FABNO

Naturopathic Specialists

When patterns are broken, new worlds emerge.
TULI KUPFERBERG

"I believe communication is a modality of healing. If doctors don't communicate with their patients, and patients don't communicate with their doctors, it is difficult to move toward healing."

Daniel Rubin, a board-certified naturopathic oncologist and founding president of the Oncology Association of Naturopathic Physicians, is passionate about his work—and he communicates it well. "We empower people through our intention, which is to communicate with and educate them about their disease. We're very upbeat here. We do everything we can to empower our patients." Dr. Rubin is one of six doctors at Scottsdale-based Naturopathic Specialists, and his expertise—and the only thing he's ever done—is naturopathic oncology. But that doesn't mean he's isolated from medical doctors. Indeed, he has deliberately inserted himself within the traditional medical community in Scottsdale, perceiving that he helps more people by being a part of the medical community.

Dr. Rubin has earned accolades from the medical community by attending meetings at the Scottsdale Healthcare Tumor Boards. "It took me two years to gain attendance into their meetings. I enjoy being there because I want the doctors to understand that naturopaths have specialties that can complement the work they themselves are doing."

The relationship is working. Medical or radiation oncologists direct about 30 percent of their patients to Dr. Rubin—something rarely heard of. The rest of his patients are made up of self-referrals or community referrals; a portion of those patients choose to do nothing but nonconventional approaches to heal their cancer.

Treatments vary by cancer type, but Dr. Rubin tends to focus on the molecular aspect of the disease. "I want to know what makes cancer tick. In general, I treat patients according to a methodology. I attempt to get to know the physiological behavior of the tumor and how it translates into something that we spot in the urine or blood. We then compare this to the diagnosis, in addition to the person's symptoms and their other health challenges. From that basis, we develop a treatment plan.

"I also look at inflammatory pathways. I'm a steward of the

inflammatory aspects of oncology, the clotting pathways, the inability of wounds to heal, and how this relates to cancer, the immune pathways, insulin axis, and so on. This is the beauty of our methodology and our approach to patient care."

Inflammation is of particular interest to Dr. Rubin, as he perceives that many cancers present themselves as unhealed wounds. "Colon cancer is an example of this theory. There seems to be a constant invocation of the wound healing cascade, which sets the stage for the growth of cells—in this case, cancer cells—and a cascade of growth that stops short of completion and then starts over again. By approaching a patient with this methodology, we can give treatments that focus on these events. In this way, patients can move toward healing as they transition to the later steps of the wound healing cascade. Movement like this can significantly and positively impact the healing of the person with cancer. There is a complex physiological basis for this, and many new cancer drugs are pointed toward these events."

Detoxification is also part of Dr. Rubin's protocol. So are dietary and lifestyle changes, which he thinks are central to the role of the naturopathic physician. "That's why NDs are such a good complement to the entire care team, because we bring a unique style and approach to each person's case."

Communication, education, empowerment, natural remedies, nutritional supplements, and, at times, intravenous and injections of medicine go into his elixir of treatments. I asked Dr. Rubin how he sees the connection between mental attitude and healing. "The mental/emotional status of the patient can create physiology that becomes ubiquitous in the body. It makes a huge difference. I recognize the value of the oneness between the mind and body, and we do teach creative visualization at the clinic. Mostly though, we offer unintentional mind-body therapy because we work so closely with our patients. Our staff is involved with and supports patients with so many of their decisions."

Like most NDs, Dr. Rubin's modalities include acupuncture,

homeopathics, and "things that access the vital force," so he can treat the side effects of chemotherapy and radiation while boosting their potential curative impact. "I want to positively affect the paradigm of oncology by bringing as much naturopathic medicine as possible to as many people as possible. That's why I appreciate working with allopathic physicians. The way to help the most number of people is through integrative medicine."

Part of Dr. Rubin's educational philosophy is that "Cancer is to a tumor as an allergy is to a runny nose. For instance you can take an antihistamine, and the symptom (runny nose) will go away. But the allergy persists." In short, Dr. Rubin is suggesting that if we remove a tumor, we may not be addressing the core issue of the cancer.

He concludes by illuminating the intrinsic partnership between himself and his patients: "The great deeds in medicine come from raw physician talent embraced by the unwavering courage of our patients."

The Particulars

Where: Scottsdale, Arizona, a suburb of Phoenix.

Who: Six physicians, six nurses, a manager, and multiple supporting staff members.

What to expect: Dr. Rubin explains, "When people call our clinic, they will speak to our new-patient coordinator or to the clinic manager. We believe the decision to undergo treatment from a particular physician is an important choice. We also understand the difficulties and stresses that people with cancer undergo and how critical the decisions they make can be. For these reasons, we give our prospective patients as much time as they need to ask preliminary questions before they come to see our physicians. By the time they get to our clinic, they feel confident in their decision, and so we have more time to go over their case and create treatment plans."

Typical routine: "When people get to our clinic, they can expect to have a great experience. Our staff members are caring and fun, and they take pride in their jobs. They are there to help patients in any way they can, and we always go that extra step. We often have out-of-town guests/patients at our clinic, and our staff is certainly there to help with trip planning and accommodations. Before a patient arrives from out of town, we make sure that their appointments have already been scheduled, so that when they arrive, they can start treatment right away. Oftentimes, we order laboratory tests before patients even arrive so we can get a good jump start on their case. Patients meet with the doctor, and thereafter, that physician will create, confirm, or modify the treatment plan. The patient is also supplied a typed document of the treatment plan, and all information from their chart is available to them. We have no secrets, and we believe that patients are active participants in their own care team."

Where to stay: "We do not provide lodging at our clinic, as we provide outpatient services only. We have unique relationships with many top hotels in the local area and can aid patients in obtaining special rates."

Cost: "Naturopathic Specialists does not take insurance, but we will provide the paperwork necessary for patients to submit to their provider. We are unable to accept Medicare. You may call the clinic and discuss costs; office-visit fees are fixed, but treatment costs vary."

Contact Information:

Dr. Daniel Rubin
Naturopathic Specialists, LLC
7331 East Osborn Drive, Suite 330
Scottsdale, AZ 85251
480-990-1111
naturopathicspecialists.com

Do not be too timid and squeamish about your actions. All life is an experiment.
RALPH WALDO EMERSON

ABRAM HOFFER, MD, PHD

Orthomolecular Therapy
Author of *Healing Cancer: Complementary Vitamin & Drug Treatments,* with Dr. Linus Pauling

Life loves to be taken by the lapel and told: "I'm with you kid. Let's go."
MAYA ANGELOU

I interviewed Dr. Abram Hoffer about a week before he died at age ninety-two. I detected nothing to suggest that he was ill or weak, although his son later told me that he was not at all well. Even so, his voice was strong, his conviction deep, and his desire to continue his work unyielding. In fact, at the end of our conversation, he told me to include an invitation to readers to visit him at his office in Canada anytime, saying "walk-ins welcome."

His open-door policy represented what I clearly perceived as an open-heart policy, one where healing patients was far more important than conforming to the status quo.

***

"Let's be honest," Dr. Abram Hoffer said, "we know almost nothing about cancer. We have theories. There are many alternative treatments, but they're all based on theories because all the research is going into drugs. It's all mixed up."

The mix-up he was referring to is the conventional medical system that governs the treatment of cancer and other diseases in the United States and in Canada. Based in Victoria, British Columbia, Dr. Hoffer was no fool when it came to medicine. He graduated from the University of Saskatchewan in Saskatoon with a BSA and an MSA. He then went on to the University of Minnesota to get his PhD in nutrition, then to the University of Toronto, where he earned his MD. He specialized in psychiatry and became the director of psychiatric research for the Saskatchewan Department of Public Health and an associate professor of medicine at the University of Saskatchewan. He penned more than five hundred peer-reviewed and popular articles, and more than thirty academic and popular books. With this record, he was entitled to his opinion about the myopic and narrow-minded medical protocol practiced in North America.

"The medical profession today is a mess. It's been taken over by drug companies. They're controlling medical research, and their principal concern is to make money," he said with conviction. "Any new ideas take about fifty years to get accepted."

However, according to Dr. Hoffer, that's more of a tradition than a new problem. He illustrated his point by citing that when the stethoscope was first invented, it was rejected because it was considered indecent to place the instrument on a female's chest. When anesthesia was introduced, it was also rejected because the puritanical atmosphere of the day claimed that "God said women are supposed to suffer when in childbirth."

"These are classic examples of how new ideas have a terrible time gaining acceptance," Dr. Hoffer explained. "These days, because the drug companies are controlling what doctors do, the idea of vitamin therapy for cancer and other diseases is typically rejected."

The angry tone in his voice was understandable given that the mainstream medical community generally does not recognize his work.

Even so, the results he saw for a variety of conditions, including cancer, using a nutritional approach known as Orthomolecular Therapy (OMT) were very promising.

In 1955, while practicing in Saskatchewan, Dr. Hoffer and his colleagues discovered that niacin (B3) lowers cholesterol. At the time, Dr. Hoffer, working with his close colleague Dr. Humphry Osmond, began treating acute schizophrenic patients with large quantities of niacin and vitamin C and witnessed significant and positive results. At first, his work was published in highly regarded peer-reviewed scientific journals, but largely ignored. Then Dr. Hoffer's work became highly controversial, especially after the Nobel-winning chemist Linus Pauling publically endorsed it and called for research into nutritional therapies for major mental illnesses.

In the fall of 2008, Dr. Hoffer's innovative work with niacin was supported by a study at Johns Hopkins University. Brains from deceased schizophrenics (but not other people) were found to have diminished expression of receptors for niacin. This suggests that schizophrenic brains may not respond as well as those of other people to normal doses of niacin.

"I'd been claiming all along that large doses of niacin would make them better. Now we have some proof," Dr. Hoffer exclaimed.

Obviously, it takes time for the research to filter down to the classroom, but Dr. Hoffer was distressed that his work had not been taken seriously in the past. If it had, doctors would now be administering nutritionally oriented treatments as a regular practice.

Unexpectedly, his work with schizophrenia is what alerted him to how OMT could successfully treat cancer. In 1960, he was treating a schizophrenic patient who also had lung cancer. As the treatment progressed, not only was the schizophrenia rapidly and successfully managed, but the doctor who was treating the cancer said that the tumor was also diminishing. Three months later, the patient was doing well. When Dr. Hoffer had first started treating him with OMT, the man had been given about a month to live.

Shortly after his success with the lung cancer patient, Dr. Hoffer treated a young woman with a highly malignant sarcoma on her arm. She was scheduled to have surgery to remove the arm when Dr. Hoffer suggested she try the niacin treatment for a month. She agreed, and her surgeon conceded to holding off on the surgery. One month later, the cancer was gone.

Eventually, other cancer patients came to Dr. Hoffer for OMT treatment, which he gladly administered. The three dominant vitamins that make up his protocol are vitamins C, D, and B3.

In the late 1960s, Dr. Hoffer began working with Linus Pauling, who by then was an acclaimed scientist. Pauling and his colleague Ewan Cameron were successfully treating cancer with vitamin C, producing groundbreaking results. But *The New England Journal of Medicine* had a different point of view. It printed that the Mayo Clinic had conducted several prospective, double-blind studies to test Pauling and Cameron's claims. The studies concluded that Pauling's findings were based on "improper statistic analysis of data from a case series." According to Dr. Hoffer's autobiography, Pauling insisted that the Mayo Clinic studies did not use the same method of administering the vitamins, and thus, had different outcomes. Pauling subsequently wrote a rebuttal to the damning article, but the *Journal* did not publish it.

Fueled by conviction, the two men worked together in an attempt to document and track the success of their patients, with the hopes of getting the data published in a mainstream journal. They also collaborated on writing mass-market books about their discoveries. Although they met with ridicule and resistance from the medical community, Dr. Hoffer was successful in creating and editing what's now called *The Journal of Orthomolecular Medicine*(orthomed.org/index.html). In this journal, Dr. Hoffer published 131 reports and forty-eight editorials, accurately shedding light on the substantial impact of OMT.

These days, open-minded conventional medical doctors, in addition to alternative and naturopathic practitioners, recognize and use OMT as part of their cancer treatment. "I've seen fifty thousand people through the years," claimed Hoffer. "I've seen the worst get well. Many people who were dying of cancer have had their lives prolonged."

Dr. Hoffer presented a philosophical view of what was behind the resistance to accepting the promising results. "If you have a million people saying the earth is flat and only a few who say it's not, those few will not be accepted."

When asked about well-meaning MDs who would relish the idea of a kinder, less brutal treatment for cancer, Dr. Hoffer replied, "Medical doctors either don't know about OMT or have been told it's ineffective. They're brainwashed in medical schools, and the students end up content because they believe that what they're taught is the only way to do medicine."

My own experience reflects what Dr. Hoffer claimed. When I was talking with my oncologist after my first diagnosis, I asked him about vitamin C therapy. He took a deep breath, shifted his weight, and simply said, "I don't agree with Linus Pauling. I just don't agree that it works." That was the end of the conversation.

Just like chemo, radiation, surgery, and other conventional treatments, sometimes OMT doesn't work either. "There are so many ways to look at things from a scientific point of view," Dr. Hoffer told me. "We have ideas on why it works for some people, but we're not sure. We know it increases antioxidants. We know that the oxygen in our bodies tends to get burned up unless we have ample amounts of vitamins C and E and other minerals. But some of it also has to do with the conviction that it *can* work."

This was consistent with the observations of the other doctors I've interviewed for this book. We're being asked to believe in something we've been told doesn't work, and we're talking about the issue of hope.

Dr. Hoffer gave two examples. "In about 2002, there was a woman who had kidney cancer. It had spread around her aorta, and she was given six months to live. They literally told her to write her will. She was in hospice when I put her on vitamin C, which gave her hope. Two years later, the hospice called me and said a miracle had occurred, because there was no more tumor. Every year, we get a postcard from this patient telling us how she's doing, and she's doing well.

"There's another case that comes to mind, a man who had throat cancer. I gave him OMT once or twice, that's all. I didn't see him again for five years. Then he popped in to see me. We chatted. He was moving to Mexico to start a new business. At last he looked at me and said, 'Do you know what helped me more than anything else? When you put your hand on my shoulder and told me I was going to make it.'

"Hope is a critical part of any treatment. Good doctors know this. They'll give the patient hope without even thinking about it. If you go to a doctor, and he says you'll be dead in six months, get out of there and never go back. See your situation as a challenge, not a death sentence. Say to yourself, 'Let's see what we'll do to get through this.'"

Dr. Hoffer agreed that there's a relationship between the mind and body. Since he is a psychiatrist, that view is not a surprise; but rather than preaching to his patients about this dynamic, he's created a model that he believes supports their healing and wellness. "If you come to me, there are four things I do: First, I make sure you have shelter. You can't be living on the streets and get better. Next, I make sure you have proper nutrition. If you don't eat well, your condition won't improve. Then I treat you with civility and humanity. That includes giving you hope, encouragement, and advice. Finally, I offer you the best possible treatment I can. It may include conventional treatment, but it will absolutely include vitamins and minerals in the right doses."

Dr. Hoffer said the "right dose" is unique to each patient, and it doesn't mean going to the health food store and buying more Cs. OMT is often administered intravenously, so it's important to use the services of a skilled health care professional. "It's trial and error," he admitted. "If we had a reasonable medical system, there'd be extensive research on this, and we would know the best quality and quantity to use."

Still, Dr. Hoffer was glad to report that there is a growing international movement to study and use OMT. The University of Kansas, for example, has an OMT component in its medical school. Some newly published papers are beginning to validate how valuable it is. Vitamin C therapy for ovarian cancer is especially effective, and Dr. Hoffer reported that the medical exams at University of Kansas are now referring to the use of OMT.

"There is some good research that's proving that vitamins B3 and D3—in addition to vitamin C—could prevent cancer. But you have to balance all these vitamins in the right doses, so you must work with someone who knows the chemistry of all this."

Changing the current cancer culture to include more research and use of OMT will require outcry and demand from patients, he told me. "People need to read books and educate themselves. Make noise. Get the attention of presidents. We're all going broke because of the cost of drugs. We have to teach each other about other options. We're all responsible for what's happened. It's up to us to change it."

To learn more about OMT or to find a practitioner who can administer OMT, go to the International Society of Orthomolecular Medicine (ISOM) at ort homed.org. You can also read a paper by Dr. Hoffer, entitled "Clinical Procedures in Treating Terminally Ill Cancer Patients with Vitamin C" (ortho med.org/resources/papers/hofcanc.htm) . To find a list of his other books and articles, see the appendix.

None will improve your lot
If you yourselves do not.
BERTOLT BRECHT

CHAPTER 10

Faith

There can be no happiness if the things
we believe in are different from the
things we do.
FREYA STARK

After a cancer diagnosis, many people turn to faith to carry them through the fear and hardship. I've been in awe of and marveled at the people I interviewed and the diversity of where they place their faith. It drives home the point that you don't *have* to believe in God, Jesus, Moses, Mohammad, or Buddha to heal. You don't *have* to change your diet, meditate, or exercise to heal. You don't *have* to undergo chemotherapy, radiation, or surgery to heal. But there does seem to be a consistent thread in everyone I've encountered who has healed: they placed a positive faith in *something* and, by doing so, transcended disease.

Faith of any kind is powerful and pure. It is our ability to believe in something—whether Tamoxifen or transcendental meditation—even when we aren't sure how or if it will work. By definition, faith is rooted in mystery and uncertainty. But we give ourselves to it anyway and let go of trying to control the situation. That act alone—releasing resistance—clears the way for healing energy to come forth.

The placebo effect is an intriguing display of the power of faith. Thousands of compelling stories have been reported about people cured of just about everything, including cancer, from taking a substance that had no medical properties. Even so, symptoms receded, in some cases to the point of clearing up entirely, because of the faith people had in the mock drugs.

This is the power of our mind, our faith. It's our own innate power.

It's essential that we recognize where we place our faith. If we believe that we are not worthy of success, that we are not worth loving, that our dreams will never come true, that we are stuck and can't leave a marriage or job that brings us misery, that we have no power or voice, that life is not worth living, and that a cancer diagnosis is synonymous with death, then we are placing our faith in limitations, contraction, restriction, and doubt. Ultimately, we are placing our faith in the power of fear and decline. That's as good as saying, "Life is a brutal and meaningless event. No matter what I do, nothing works out. I'm not sure how or why it works that way, but I have faith that there are forces waging against me and everything will fall apart." And so they do.

If, on the other hand, we believe we are worthy of being, doing, and having everything we've ever dreamed; that we are absolutely lovable and loved; that we can leave any situation that doesn't serve us because we trust that we'll be safe and that something better will replace it; that we have power beyond our comprehension; and that we have a strong and important voice; that life—with all of its ups and downs—is an adventure of magnificent proportion; and that a cancer diagnosis can be an awakening to the truth, beauty, and power of who we really are and what life is really about, then we are placing our faith in the generative power of love and evolution. That's as good as saying, "Even though life can be deeply painful, it's still a miraculous and worthwhile journey that somehow, some way, balances out. I'm not sure how or why it works that way, but I have faith that there are forces at play that are helping and guiding me, and that things always work out." And so they do.

When people speak of faith, they are typically referring to religion or spiritualiy. There is a broader faith, however, that plays out in our everyday decisions. Where we invest our faith can determine the course of our lives.

Faith is intensely personal. There isn't a one-size-fits-all package. Each of us has the right and freedom to choose where we invest our faith. When we invest our faith in a loving—rather than a random, wrathful, or vengeful—universe, we learn that we are not alone. In fact, when our hearts are open to receiving and our faith is steady, we are supported in unfathomable ways.

We are the source of our own experience, we are the master of it, we can handle it, and we are greater than it.
DAVID HAWKINS

SUSAN'S STORY

When I dare to be powerful, to use my strength in the service of my vision, then it becomes less and less important whether I am afraid.
AUDRE LORDE

Susan has an easy laugh. When I spoke with her, she was vacationing at a ski resort with her two teenaged kids and was planning to take on the challenge of some black-diamond runs.

"Sometimes my kids find it hard to believe I'm doing this well," she said with a bittersweet chuckle, "but miracles follow me around, so I'm just fine."

That wasn't the case in July 2007, when she discovered a lump in her breast. Her doctor reported that it was stage 2B breast cancer, requiring a mastectomy followed by an intensive protocol of chemo and radiation. A second opinion confirmed the diagnosis. She wanted time to think, but felt pressured to make a quick decision by the two doctors she was considering using for treatment. In her mind, they were a little too eager to "close the deal."

"At one of the doctor's offices, I saw a graph of how many breast cancer cases they take on. It reminded me of being at a car lot and seeing how they chart their sales. I panicked. I was overwhelmed with fear and wanted more time, but both doctors kept calling me about scheduling surgery and treatments."

Susan finally chose her doctor, had the surgery, and then followed up with chemo and radiation for eleven months. But by April 2008, she was experiencing excruciating pain in her back and predicted that it was more cancer.

"My doctor didn't want to do a scan, saying that everyone has backaches. But instead of bending to her point of view, I listened to my intuition and spoke up. They finally took some pictures. Sure enough, there was a tumor on my spine, and after a PET scan, they found it had metastasized to my thigh, iliac, and hip bones. They call all of that stage 4 breast cancer."

The news was devastating. Susan and her boyfriend wanted information: they wanted to know what to expect, and they wanted to know Susan's options. Her oncologist concurred and called in a specialist for a meeting. In the meeting, the doctors admitted that the spinal tumor was visible in the scans from 2007, but had been overlooked. Now Susan would need more radiation to treat the mass on her spine, and the treatment would leave a hole in her vertebrae. The doctors' solution was a procedure to fill the hole with cement.

It was all too much to grasp. "I had to get out of there," Susan recalled. She and her boyfriend left speechless.

A few days later, they visited another doctor. "My boyfriend finally said, 'Speak to us straight!' That's when the doctor said, 'Statistically speaking, you have three to five years to live.' She then walked me through what she seemed to think was a sure and predictable demise. I was completely stunned and realized there was no way I could work with a doctor who gave me a false sense of hopelessness. We left there having no idea what to do next."

The gloomy prognosis led to the next big blow: Susan's boyfriend left her. He couldn't cope. She understood intellectually, but suddenly, in addition to having metastasized cancer, she was alone.

Even though Susan had spent her life being self-sufficient and independent, this was too much to bear by herself. She grew up taking care of herself and, up to that point, had relied on no one but herself. This man who was now leaving her was one of only a handful of people she had trusted. Now she was alone, and everything caved in.

In that moment, Susan began to think she should put her faith in a higher source. After all, the scientific "facts" were feeding her nothing but a fear so intense it made her physically sick. "I had a meltdown, mentally, physically, and spiritually. I couldn't get out of bed. I wasn't sure God existed. I kept asking where he was, why had he forsaken me. It was a very dark time."

Soon after, she called her old friend Ginny. "Instinctively, I knew I could trust her. I hadn't been in contact with her for three or four years, but she was who I called. I was totally honest and said, 'I'm in trouble. I gotta come see you. I'm having horrible thoughts. I don't know what to do. I'm hopeless.'"

Ginny was participating in some programs at the Chautauqua Institution in New York (ciweb.org) and urged Susan to join her there. Chautauqua, Ginny explained, is a retreat center where music, writing, art, dance, recreation, health, and spirituality are celebrated in a variety of forms and ideologies. Ginny would provide Susan with a bed, and she promised Susan that the environment at Chautauqua would be very nurturing.

"When I arrived, I was totally broken. Ginny was right there for me and, after getting me some tea, took me to a healing service. We entered a small cottage chapel, and they performed an anointing healing ceremony on me with holy oils. They prayed over me. A red-haired woman, who had been knitting by herself in the room, knelt down in front of me and recited Psalm 23. We prayed together, and it was very powerful. I had no idea who these people were, but they were praying for me. I was crying, and my heart began to heal. I began to understand that I was not alone. I felt the power of prayer and the grace of God transforming me. I finally felt a nanosecond of peace."

Psalm 23 (King James Version)

The Lord is my shepherd; I shall not want.

He maketh me to lie down in green pastures: he leadeth me beside the still waters.

He restoreth my soul: he leadeth me in the paths of righteousness for his name's sake.

Yea, though I walk through the valley of the shadow of death, I will fear no evil: for thou art with me; thy rod and thy staff they comfort me.

Thou preparest a table before me in the presence of mine enemies: thou anointest my head with oil; my cup runneth over.

Surely goodness and mercy shall follow me all the days of my life: and I will dwell in the house of the Lord for ever.

"Several days later, I was walking on the campus when the same red-haired woman approached me. 'I've been looking all over for you!' she said. She presented me with a beautiful prayer shawl that she had been knitting for six months and that twenty-eight people had prayed over. She didn't know who she would give it to, but after meeting me, she finally knew where it would go.

"That night, I slept with the shawl covering my body. I felt a healing presence in the shawl. Love infiltrated me. I awoke the next morning to find the cross that had been stitched onto it was resting right on my tumor site."

In the four days she stayed at Chautauqua, Susan experienced deep healing. But as she hugged Ginny good-bye, she realized she had arrived at a crossroads. "I told Ginny that I had to find a doctor who could treat my whole being, not just the physical symptoms and the problems related to the cancer. My medical experience up until then made me unsure I would find a doctor like that, but I prayed and asked to be led. At that point, my faith went from dabbling with a relationship with Jesus to aligning my life with his love and guidance. I knew I had to either transform my life or give in to the demise predicted by my previous doctor."

When Susan got home, she embraced the purple shawl, reminded of the beauty of her experience at the healing ceremony. As she recalled her time there, it awakened feelings within her that God *was* present and that she had not been abandoned. "I knew I could believe in God's grace and his unconditional love for me. I started talking to him. I said, 'You've ripped me to shreds, but I'm going to trust that you're here with me. And I'm going to sit down with this Bible every day. And Jesus, I've heard you're a healer. You're the great physician. You've worked miracles. Well, I'm done, and I give my will over to you. Please, please work miracles for me.'"

From that moment on, Susan was true to her vow. Every morning before her children awoke, she'd wrap herself in the shawl, sit in her "prayer chair," light a candle, and read passages from the Bible. Psalm 46, with the line "Be still and know that I am" resonated with her. She spent as much time as she could reciting it and sitting in silence with God.

"I live in an old church rectory, and I can see the cross through the window from my chair. I began writing down scriptures that spoke to me. I heard the wisdom, guidance, and discernment present in Jesus's healing. Every day, I read the Bible, and I prayed and wrote down passages. Wisdom is more precious than silver and gold. I was guided back to believing that miracles are real. They do happen. I started to believe it and know it. I felt it on a gut level. I prayed every day, and pretty soon miracles began to happen to me."

Susan's son was attending a Catholic school. Occasionally, she'd enter the simple school chapel, where a single, carved, wooden image of Jesus hung over the altar, and she'd pray. Usually, she'd close her eyes and pray before the carving, but one morning her eyes remained opened as she stared at the image. To Susan, it was stunningly beautiful. She wept and asked Jesus to let her know that he was with her, and then she had an epiphany.

"I prayed that he was going to heal me, that he'd walk with me through this journey and give me back my strength. I cried, and I prayed. Then this pink glow came over the sculpture of Jesus and enveloped it. There was about two feet of this pink glow all the way around it. I couldn't take my eyes off it. Then the image of Christ began to morph into an androgynous figure, from man to woman to man to woman again, and I realized that Jesus was and is the image of all of us—man and woman—all of us! It was amazing!

"I brought someone else in to see it, and I saw it again right there, the pink glowing Jesus in the dark little chapel. But the person with me didn't see it."

Susan knew then that this was her personal journey. Elated, she left the chapel and walked the school grounds. October leaves scattered about her feet. She headed to a park bench, where she saw a few chestnuts on the ground. "I like chestnuts, so I picked up the ones I could see. Then I wanted more. Playfully, I said, 'God, I would really love to find more chestnuts.' Twenty seconds later, the wind picked up, and I was bombarded by chestnuts. I had this very clear feeling inside that said, 'Do not struggle to look for jewels. Ask and I will send them to you in abundance.' Since then, I've experienced miracle after miracle. I wear a bracelet made of chestnuts, and I sent every one of my friends a chestnut."

Guided by faith and trust, Susan began researching her options and discovered that there were indeed medical professionals who practiced integrative oncology. She went to Boston and attended a symposium put on by the Institute of Coaching at McLean Hospital. There Susan met the founder of the Institute, Margaret Moore, who offered to be her coach.

Margaret helped her to define her goals and encouraged her to look for new doctors and treatment plans.

Susan then attended a meeting in New York given by the Society for Integrative Oncologists. In a room filled with hundreds of doctors and professionals, she took a turn at the microphone during the question-and-answer period. She wept and told her story, sharing her perspective about what it was like to be a cancer patient and the impact of cancer treatments. "The community embraced me and invited me to join them for dinner. By divine coincidence, I ended up at the same table as a doctor I had researched and wanted to work with. My prayers were answered, and he is still my doctor today."

Susan now works with integrative oncologists as a patient representative so that future patients can have a better cancer-care experience.

As she treated her physical body, she continued to grow her spiritual commitment. Her friend Ginny planted the idea of assembling an active prayer community through a weekly teleconference that would allow people to support her by participating in her healing. Once a week, Susan wraps herself in the purple shawl, lights a candle, and pulls out her Bible, and friends and family from all over the country call a toll-free number and talk. These calls are a "sacred gathering place," where Susan relays what's going on in her life and with her treatment. She asks for prayers from callers, and they read Bible passages and offer other spiritual insights. Then she lies down. Everyone on the call closes their eyes and visualizes putting their hands on Susan's body. They send her love, support, and healing. They pray aloud, offer words of encouragement, and imagine their healing hands on her body for fifteen minutes. This happens every week.

"I can feel it in my body," Susan said with delight, "on a cellular level. I now understand that faith heals and will cure my cancer. Doubts may come back, but I quickly get back into the chair, into the Bible; throw the shawl over myself; and remember all the miracles that have come to me. And the doubts disappear."

After only six months, PET scans revealed that one of her tumors was completely gone, while all the others had diminished by half. She did undergo radiation for the tumor in her spine, which left her in pain and with fragile bones. Now she no longer experiences back pain and is off all medications. She continues to sit in her prayer chair with the warmth of the purple shawl surrounding her as she prays and reads the Bible each morning.

This spiritual devotion has led Susan to an emotional freedom she'd never known before. "Those toxic thoughts of despair that once paralyzed me are now merely nanoseconds of anxiety and are quickly dispelled by God. I don't have to work toward God; God comes to me—if I can be still. *Be still and know that I am God* is my mantra. There is no need to perform or do or be perfect in order to receive the love God offers. I have been transformed from within after trying for so long to transform myself from the outside."

Susan credits her relationship with Christ for her sustenance. "My story now is my spiritual life. The narrative of my past I see as purposeful and full of meaning, as are all the experiences, stories, and events that led me here. My journey is no longer about cancer. All that matters is living each day to the fullest, based on all that God is teaching me. Regret is living in the past. Fear is living in the future. But hope always resides in the present."

No one is required to have faith like Susan's in order to negotiate black-diamond ski slopes. But my bet is that she handles them with grace.

Susan has started a non-profit organization that guides people on how to create prayer lines. For more information, please visit prayershawl.org.

Keep your heart with all diligence, for out of it are the issues of life.
PROVERBS 4:23

LARRY DOSSEY, MD

Prayer, Miracles, and Remote Healing

Author of *Prayer Is Good Medicine: How to Reap the Healing Benefits of Prayer*

Our real blessings often appear to us in the shape of pains, losses, and disappointments, but let us have patience, and we soon shall see them in their proper figures.
JOSEPH ADDISON

Having read some of Dr. Larry Dossey's eleven books, and especially after speaking with him, I think he's pretty much the perfect example of a man with a sharp, inquisitive, scientific mind, coupled with an open heart that's driven by insatiable curiosity about how we as spiritual beings influence the physical matter we occupy.

Trained as an internist and practicing medicine since 1974, Dr. Dossey is fascinated by the as-of-yet undiscovered science that may someday explain what we call miracle healings. Fueled by this fascination, Dr. Dossey has devoted decades to studying and writing about how prayer specifically and spirituality in general impact our physical well-being.

"We know that there's a relationship between our thoughts and our bodies," Dr. Dossey said. "That stuff is already integrated into medicine. What's more interesting to me is that our thoughts can affect *other people's* cells! This is important for anyone with an illness. It means that healing influences can operate remotely—from a distance—coming from other people, for your benefit. If someone sends you compassionate, positive thoughts through a prayer, it can make a difference. That means you don't have to carry the whole burden of getting well yourself." The science backing his claims is illustrated throughout his books, especially in *Healing Words: The Power of Prayer and the Practice of Medicine.*

He then recited the story of the wife of a fundamentalist Christian minister who was diagnosed with cervical cancer. Her surgeon suggested that she have a hysterectomy, but instead her husband organized a prayer meeting at their church. "She reported to me that when the prayer meeting took place, she felt, for the first time in her life, an amazing sensation of heat come over her body, and she knew she was healed," recalled Dr. Dossey. "This woman wasn't crazy. She was very bright, and she knew she was healed.

"After the healing session, she asked her surgeon to do another biopsy prior to the operation, but he refused. In her heart, she knew a healing had occurred, so she told him that she wouldn't do the surgery unless he consented to another test. He gave in, and much to his surprise, the cancer was gone."

Then there's the story of Rita Klaus, one of Dr. Dossey's favorites. Rita didn't have cancer, but she did have a crippling case of multiple sclerosis. "Rita depended on crutches or a wheelchair to get around. One day, her husband took her to a healing meeting. She reported the same kind of warm, loving sensation washing over her. Days passed, and nothing else happened until she dreamed that the Virgin Mary came to her and said, 'Just ask for the healing.' When she awoke, she did just that, and a few days later, she got well. This woman went from being a complete cripple to running around doing normal activities."

In a book she wrote, called *Rita's Story*, she reports that some of her doctors shared the joy of her recovery, while others were actually angered by the healing.[1] One doctor accused her of having a twin sister who had been ill and said that Rita was a fraud. Dr. Dossey said, "That kind of attitude is a refuge for doctors who aren't prepared to accept this type of thing. But these kinds of healings happen all the time. And I believe they are the natural order of things, or they wouldn't happen at all. Science doesn't yet have all the laws of nature figured out. We're ignorant of what triggers that type of healing, but it's still part of the natural order."

Recalling how other people have told me that their doctors either didn't want to know about their recovery or became hostile because of it, I asked why MDs are so threatened by mystery healings. Dr. Dossey explained that docs are trained to learn and treat by the laws of science, and they believe these so-called miraculous healings defy those laws. When the laws of science are bypassed, it can make them very uncomfortable.

"I get criticized by skeptics who don't want to hear about this, but I reject that totally. These people are usually logically, analytically, and scientifically oriented and may be agnostic. However, I don't want to be too hard on doctors," he continued. "Even in my own medical training, I was told that these types of healing are rare and that we'd probably never see anything like them throughout our entire practice. Yet that's not true. These cases occur in practically every disease you can imagine."

He quickly pointed out that no single protocol brings about healing, and there are, in fact, plenty of cases full of contradictions. "Take the guy who had lung cancer and was given only a few weeks to live. He decided that if that were the case, he was going to do what he loved the most, which was to smoke. So he increased his habit from two to four packs a day, and still the cancer went away.

"I've spent a long time chasing down so-called spontaneous remissions. It's darn hard to come up with any common pathway in terms of the technique that people choose to get well."

In the book *Remarkable Recovery: What Extraordinary Healings Tell Us About Getting Well and Staying Well,* written by Caryle Hirshberg and Marc Ian Barasch, the authors provide stories of people who experienced healing.[2] "The book gives guidelines about what people do to set the stage for these incredible turnarounds," Dr. Dossey explained. "Sixty or so people were interviewed about what they thought was responsible for their recovery from cancer. They attributed it to all kinds of things. Some fought it; others accepted it—in equal numbers. Some said healing was because of prayer; some emphasized singing or taking up a hobby, walking, exercising, or learning a new art or craft. You look at this list, and you scratch your head, saying, 'Wait a minute. What's the common thread here?'

"It's really up to everyone to ask themselves if there is a common pathway. I would be hesitant to formulate a specific behavioral pattern that sets the stage for a cure."

To Dr. Dossey, the answer could lie in the place where science and spirituality intersect. "Science and spirituality are very interactive," he said. "Even the medical schools are starting to understand that. The mention of spirituality used to be a bunch of mumbo jumbo in the medical field. But that day has passed. You can't get out of med school now without proving that you can take a spiritual history on patients. As part of their certification, hospitals must now assess the spiritual health of their patients. That's because spirituality is a respectable player in healing. And there's a lot of science to back that up." According to Dr. Dossey, in 1993 only three of the 125 medical schools in the US offered course work in spirituality. Now more than ninety of them do.

Enthusiasm aside, Dr. Dossey admitted that relying on prayer and spirituality for a cure isn't absolute. "People condemn prayer healing because it isn't always effective, but penicillin doesn't work for everyone either. People tend to let conventional therapy off the hook even though only about 75 percent of what doctors do meets the empirical standard of proof. My point is that we should be open to anything that works, whether it's conventional or not."

The good news for those who believe in the power of faith, prayer, and other types of spiritual application is that the science behind these intangible forces is becoming clearer to our logical minds. "There's overwhelming evidence that spirituality has a significant impact on health in general. Studies show that if you adopt some sort of spiritual approach—and commit to it—it doesn't appear to matter greatly which approach you take. If it becomes part of your belief system and you integrate it into your life, on average you'll live longer and have fewer illnesses.

"In essence, spirituality favors health. One analysis shows that spiritually active people live seven to thirteen years longer than people who are not spiritually committed. Even if you stop smoking, you don't get that big of a gain. Medical schools are starting to recognize this.

"If you look at individual cases, you can find stunning examples of people whose spiritual beliefs seemed to set the stage for spontaneous remission. These are some of the most sensational remissions you can imagine. Even though spiritual commitment is no guarantee, there is no question that belief systems, faith, and reliance on a transcendent power can set the stage for spontaneous healings, even involving cancer."

As thrilling as this is, the good doctor doesn't pretend that having a spiritual life will absolutely save you from a painful death. "There's a long list of saints and mystics who died of terrible diseases. I had a correspondence with a woman who was a devout nun—very spiritually evolved—living in a convent in France. When she got a lump in her breast, she proclaimed that God would protect her. But after the biopsy came back positive, she was devastated, derailed. Here's a woman who'd spent her entire life in spiritual work. Her expectations hadn't been lived up to. Consequently, she experienced horrible shame and guilt.

"New Age guilt," claimed Dr. Dossey, "is when you think you're far enough along on the spiritual path that this kind of stuff shouldn't happen to you, or that your spiritual faith will cure you and it doesn't. It all goes to show that we simply don't know how it all works."

One thing that is certain (and truly heartening news) is that the culture among doctors is changing. Every year, Dr. Dossey is invited to speak at a Harvard-sponsored conference called Update in Internal Medicine. Hundreds of MDs come from all over the world to spend an intensive week learning about the latest developments in their field. In 2008, he spoke about miracle cures.

"I figured they'd run me off," he recalled with a chuckle. "I assembled and spoke about some of the finest cases I could. I asked why we have so much skepticism toward these things. I asked why so few of them are published in our journals even though they occur everywhere.

"I really thought it would fall flat, but to my shock the response was great. All of a sudden people were coming forward and sharing their own stories about miracle cases. It became obvious that the reason they don't talk about these things is that they are afraid or embarrassed. You know, officially these things aren't supposed to happen, but they do. So these doctors are caught in cognitive dissonance. I provided them with a safe atmosphere where they wouldn't be judged."

Dr. Dossey discussed with the doctors how physicians usually respond to unexpected healings. "When a terrible disease simply goes away, doctors often call this event 'the natural course of the disease.' But that's no explanation at all," he said. "That's like saying 'What happens, happens.'"

"I discussed how these spectacular healings are rarely written up, and when they are, the human side of the case gets left out. You wind up with a 'white female, forty-five-years old,' and so on. The description of the case is solely physical. You get no sense of the person, what they believed, and why they thought their disease went away."

Dr. Dossey emphasized the importance of getting the inside story of the people to whom these miracles occur. "Nearly all the physicians opened up and responded enthusiastically. In fact, they were hungry to tell their stories. When I told them that my next book was about premonitions, they insisted that I relay some of my personal experiences. Then they couldn't wait to tell their own. One internist said that she dreams about her patients' results—the actual numbers—before she even orders the tests. That sparked all kinds of conversation.

"A few weeks later, I gave the same talk to another group of doctors, and the same thing happened. It's amazing what comes out when they're given the right context to talk about it."

With that revelation in mind, I asked Dr. Dossey about what the future holds for the allopathic medical world. He said, "We don't have a health care system in this country; we have a disease care system. Where health care is concerned, everyone knows we're headed into a black hole. We will bankrupt the country if we continue to rely on high-tech medicine without focusing on prevention. It's a national embarrassment that nearly fifty million people don't have health insurance, and that the most common cause of personal bankruptcy is medical bills.

"Drugs and surgical procedures will still be important in allopathic medicine, and I'm glad they are there when we need them. But prevention is essential as well. Experts say that two-thirds of all cancers and three-fourths of heart disease can be prevented by behavioral and lifestyle changes, such as proper diet, nutrition, exercise, weight management, stress reduction, and so on.

"Just imagine that for a moment. If a pharmaceutical company produced a medication that could eradicate the majority of heart disease and cancer, our two major killers, it would be heralded as a miracle. It also would probably be very expensive. But preventive measures are *already* available that can accomplish this, and most of them cost nothing. All that's required are shifts in habits, routines, and beliefs.

"We must be more critical of all therapies, and we must insist that they be tested thoroughly. This includes conventional therapies *and* unconventional ones. Unfortunately, this has not been done for around two-thirds of the therapies in common use. If we recommend a therapy, we have a responsibility to prove its safety and effectiveness. Patients must demand this. When their physician recommends any therapy, they should always ask two basic questions: 'Does it work?' and 'Is it safe?'"

With the help of this pioneering and visionary man—plus a more educated population—we can finally believe that such demands will soon be answered.

To learn more about Dr. Dossey, go to dosseydossey.com/larry/default.html. For a complete list of his books, see the appendix.

The future belongs to those who believe in the beauty of their dreams.
ELEANOR ROOSEVELT

DAVID L. FELTEN, MD, PHD

Psychoneuroimmunology
Editor, *Psychoneuroimmunology*

We taste and feel and see the truth.
We do not reason ourselves into it.
WILLIAM BUTLER YEATS

As far as Dr. David Felten is concerned, the idea that there's a connection between the mind and body is a no-brainer. More precisely, the connection is, in fact, traceable to the brain itself.

When he discovered the science behind this groundbreaking relationship, Dr. Felten was on the fast track for a career in traditional, allopathic medicine. He received his medical degree and doctorate from the University of Pennsylvania, following extensive work in neuroscience at the Massachusetts Institute of Technology (MIT) during his undergraduate education. Although he teaches extensively and has conducted hospital rounds with a neurologist in the past, Dr. Felten's heart was then, and remains now, in research.

"Until a few decades ago," he told me from Beaumont Hospitals in Royal Oak, Michigan, where he runs the research institute, "no one thought that the brain had anything to do with the immune system. No one thought that the brain regulated metabolism. In fact, when I was in med school, I was taught that the immune system is independent, autonomous, and self-regulatory."

Apparently it's not, and thanks to Dr. Felten's research, we now know that the brain is directly wired into and helps to regulate the immune system by sending it a series of ongoing neural messages. At the same time, he and others found evidence of reciprocity: the immune system also sends messages back to the brain. In essence, the brain and immune system enjoy a wonderfully reciprocal communication.

This discovery laid the foundation for a cutting-edge science known as psychoneuroimmunology, or PNI. Subsequent to his discovery and the growth of other components of PNI, Drs. Robert Ader, Nicholas Cohen, and Felten edited a two-volume textbook on the subject for researchers and medical professionals. It has been widely read and well received.

"Back in the early to mid-1980s, when I first reported the neural connections between the brain and the immune system, people said it was not possible. But my colleagues and I could show that there were nerve fibers that communicated with bone marrow, the thymus gland, the spleen, lymph nodes, and mucosa-associated lymphoid tissue. Showing that the nerves were there was step one; the next step was to prove that there was a response from the lymphoid tissue to those nerves. We identified many neurotransmitters from the nerves, and other researchers identified receptors for those neurotransmitters on target cells of the immune system. It was clear that they could signal to each other and respond to each other."

This communication raised an interesting speculation: If you're thinking that things are right with the world, are the messages to your immune system supportive and generative? And conversely, if you believe life is too hard to handle and is overwhelming and hopeless, will the brain's message to the immune system take a toll?

To elaborate on this line of inquiry, Dr. Felten cited work by Dr. John Sheridan at Ohio State University. Sheridan placed mice in a confined structure that restricted their movement. Then Sheridan challenged the mice with influenza virus. It only took only a fraction of the flu particles to create illness in mice that had been put under stress compared with mice in normal conditions. In this case, stress clearly weakened their immune systems, making them more inclined to get sick.

I asked Dr. Felten if he thought it worked the same with people. "When we showed there were connections between the brain and the immune system," he said, "we then wanted to know what parts of the brain were regulating the outflow of information to the immune system. It turns out that the hypothalamus and limbic systems, which govern emotions, behavior, reward mechanisms, and interpretation of stimuli, are responsible.

"That's when we realized there might be a functional link by which the brain can influence the immune system. If someone perceived extensive chronic stress in their life and experienced an adverse emotional reaction, then that emotion could influence the nerves that go directly to the immune system, in addition to the hormones that impact the immune system. Those stressors could alter specific components of the immune system, such as the activity of the natural killer cells that monitor cancer metastasis or take on viruses."

Stress isn't always and absolutely what causes illness, however. "Extensive research suggests that stress is not the first cause of infection; it just means that the conditions in a stressed body make it easier for the infection to occur."

Finding out you have cancer is highly stressful and could surely adversely affect the immune system, but cancer treatments leave their mark, too. Dr. Felten said that we are particularly vulnerable to the stresses that besiege us when our immune systems are weakened from challenges like chemotherapy and radiation. "If you have been going through cancer treatments or if you need surgery—which is enormously taxing on your body—then your immune system is compromised enough so that there may be a greater likelihood of metastasis. This is a situation in which I believe complementary and adjunctive therapies are very helpful. At the time of surgery, and for a long while afterward, stress management is important. Others have shown that if a patient uses guided imagery prior to surgery, it can reduce pain and result in a better outcome."

All of these progressive ideas are actually just common sense to Dr. Felten. "There are biological explanations for how the body and mind collaborate. Think of animals and how they evolved to respond to their environment. When they are injured, they respond so that they can recover. They may find a quiet place to rest and recuperate. After escaping from danger, they do not need a continuing fight-or-flight response; they need to go into a homeostatic state that allows optimum recovery, including immune recovery."

Still, the current operating system that propels our medical world uses a quick fix with drugs as the foundation for treatment, rather than exercise, stress management, good nutrition, and an environment conducive to homeostasis. Unlike animals, people tend to forget that rest and sleep are essential, not only when we are recovering, but also in our everyday lives.

"When being anxious and upset is the normal state of mind, when we drive ourselves into fight or flight 24/7, ranting and raving, engaging in contentious relationships, and exuding chronic anger, then stress hormones and fight-or-flight neural reactions get out of control. Some people have heart attacks and die in a fit of rage. It's simple physiology.

"It is very clear that certain activities help us repair and recover, such as good nutrition, exercise, and stress management. I think there is a reason that many religions have a day of rest, a Sabbath. The idea of being with family, relaxing and having downtime is very positive. It helps to control and ameliorate the stress in our lives. Rest points to another biological phenomenon. We simply cannot be on high alert all the time without paying a very expensive price physiologically."

The million-dollar question in my mind was this: does our state of mind control whether or not we get cancer? "I don't know," he answered honestly. "There is precious little evidence that a weak immune system is the primary reason why someone would acquire cancer. The external environment has a far greater influence. The strong preponderance of evidence suggests that the health of the immune system is not directly involved in the acquisition of cancer.

"However, the immune system becomes *highly* significant in regard to the growth and metastasis of cancer. A robust, natural killer-cell response and cell-mediated immunity (part of a precise acquired-immune response) appear to decrease the chance that the cancer will metastasize."

That's big news. These specific components of our immune system need to be as strong as possible after a diagnosis in order to help keep the tumor from growing or spreading. There are several simple ways to boost the immune system that Dr. Felten suggests have experimental evidence behind them: yoga, guided imagery, eating nutritiously (such as the Mediterranean diet of fish, fruits, vegetables, olive oil, and nuts), exercise, and doing whatever you can to reduce stress. This is another opportunity for complementary medicine to come into play.

I still couldn't shake the question of how we get cancer. If our immune system plays that big a role in keeping cancer from spreading, why wouldn't it also be part of the reason we get it in the first place? "There are lots of different things that may be the cause of the disease," Dr. Felten replied. "I think exposure to chemical and environmental agents, radiation, and genes that have been damaged by free radicals are part of it. But there is no single reason for cancer that we have found."

Nor is cancer a single disease. Like some other doctors I spoke to, Dr. Felten claimed that the popular cheerleading chant to "find a cure for cancer" is well intended but misleading. "Cancer is hundreds of diseases, and finding a cure will be a process of learning to regulate one cell type at a time. We will get a little better at it, then a little better, and a little bit better again.

"Breast cancer is a good example. There has been good progress, but not great. Ductal carcinoma is very common. But you may find fifty different women with fifty different sets of biomarkers expressed in and on the surface of the cancer cells. The hormonal environment of each woman may be different; their mental states may be different; their stress status may be different; their genetic machinery surely is different; and this means that each one will respond uniquely to the tumor. That's why cancer treatment is such a challenge. There is not a simple on-off switch.

"Other types of cancer, such as pancreatic, are much tougher to treat successfully. It can be less dangerous if you catch it early. If you don't, the cancer can spread and develop aggressive phenotypes that grow out of control.

"A further challenge is that in one situation you may have a patient with a stage 1, highly localized cancer with no lymph nodes involved, yet that same cancer has biomarkers and molecular expressions associated with an aggressive response. In other words, that patient might need aggressive treatment. Then you may have a patient with a more advanced stage of the same cancer that has biomarkers indicating a less aggressive course. That's where we have to get smarter. We need to look at the biomarkers early to get information on how aggressive or nonaggressive the specific cancer is—hence, individualized medicine. We also may be able to use new biomarkers to determine if a tumor (such as a head and neck cancer) will respond optimally to radiation therapy."

I like the idea of using the power of our minds to treat cancer, and I asked Dr. Felten if he thought we'd ever get to the point where PNI could treat cancer in place of chemo and radiation. He replied, "Highly unlikely. We know little about the vocabulary of neurotransmitters and hormones that influence the immune system. We know they have specific influences, but can we come up with a repertoire from the brain that is more effective than chemo? Perhaps we can learn to assist chemo or radiation therapy for better results, but it is unlikely that we can replace these approaches. Personally, I would explore pharmacological manipulation of neurotransmitters that could enable that possibility."

My dream of replacing chemo with medicinal brainwaves wasn't a fit for Dr. Felten. But what about lifestyle changes? "More than 80 percent of spending in this country is on chronic disease. We will all benefit from personally committing to exercise, good nutrition, and stress management."

This notion has been floating around for a while and has extensive scientific evidence to back it up, especially related to preventing chronic diseases. Yet until doctors start preaching the health benefits of stress management, and how it can actually help prevent chronic diseases and even protect against many forms of cancer and its spread, people probably will not pay attention because they don't think it is mainstream enough.

Dr. Felten believes we're not there yet, but we're on the way. "Medical schools are becoming more open to these preventive approaches. At Oakland University William Beaumont School of Medicine, we are integrating this approach into the platform of our curriculum. But it remains difficult to get doctors to talk with their patients about lifestyle or the science of the mind-body relationship.

"Meanwhile, everyone knows the relevance of preventative measures, but people do not take responsibility for themselves. They are drawn to instant gratification and influenced by advertisers, who convince them they need greasy, highly unhealthy fast food. Whether it is corn syrup or preservatives, high salt, bad fatty acids, or other damaging contents, if it makes money, then the manufacturers keep promoting it, and people keep buying it. While that is everyone's right in a free society, is it any wonder why our health care is so expensive? Many of the nation's chronic health care problems are partly due to wretched lifestyles."

Doctors know this, and yet (other than smoking cessation) they don't seem to be making a visible dent on their growing population of sick people. And the baby boomer generation will add to the problem simply because they are the largest of all aging populations. Emphasizing nutrition, exercise, and stress management is a simple, common-sense message to drive home to patients. Why aren't doctors doing more of it?

"Doctors have been raised with a scientific model." According to Dr. Felten, "We have to get to the genes, the core molecular mechanisms. Up until the last couple decades, we had not understood the mechanisms behind nutrition, exercise, and stress management. It was considered alternative treatment. I had a well-known doctor in medical school who criticized early use of exercise for cardiac rehabilitation. He called it 'damnable alternative medicine!'

"Remember too that doctors gain sizable amounts of their understanding of how things work through the *enormously powerful* pharmaceutical industry, especially after they finish medical school. That's how they are trained. I was at a symposium at a major medical center, at which a wonderful cardiologist was talking about the opening of a complementary medicine center, when the head of the cancer center stood up and said, 'There are three things you need to treat cancer and only three things: drugs, more drugs, and even more drugs!' That was only a little more than a decade ago."

To be sure, what we know now is a sweet omen of the promising discoveries of tomorrow. Meanwhile, thanks in part to Dr. Felten, science is finally providing evidence for the intriguing and profound idea that many people have felt intuitively for decades: our perceptions have a direct impact on our health. Since we have the power to shape our perceptions, we have the power to use our thoughts and emotions to help establish a healing internal environment. This is no longer a New Age, feel-good invention; it is a prevailing and innate tool that can help us to stay well or to heal.

Still, the term "healing" is subjective in Dr. Felten's mind. "There's a difference between being healed and being cured. I have seen people who have been healed by coming to a state of peace and understanding of the preciousness of life and the value within themselves, even if the disease takes their life. They may not have been cured, but they were healed. I have also seen people who appear to be free of cancer, but who are clearly not healed. They are still troubled and have not found peace. There's a cognitive, emotional, and spiritual process that needs to be present if they are to truly heal."

You could say that Dr. Felten's science is akin to an old saying that used to infuriate us, but which can now motivate us: it's all in your head!

Your Mind Controls You

But What Controls the Cancer Industry?

"The former director of the Chao Family Comprehensive Cancer Center at the University of California at Irvine studied how resveratrol from grape skins, a natural product, could be used as a chemotherapy agent," Dr. Felten told me with animation. "But that type of discovery will not be as profitable as a new drug, and the industry that discovers drugs is legitimately there to make a profit. They are not there to just be philanthropists. They are in business to make money for their investors and shareholders. That's what business is all about."

Most everyone in this book agrees that money—not affordable or drug-free treatment options—is what drives the medical system, keeping certain innovative breakthroughs, such as PNI, in the background.

"On the one hand, it is understandable," Dr. Felten commented. "The next generation of lipid-lowering drugs could cost billions of dollars to develop and test with clinical trials, but it's all down the drain if a bad side effect shows up."

Dr. Felten's knowledge of the drug industry surpasses that of most people I spoke with, largely because of his background as a research scientist, but also because he oversees pharmaceutical clinical trials research at Beaumont Hospitals in Michigan. Due to his position—and his unwavering integrity—he's a staunch advocate for a transparent and ethical pharmaceutical world.

"Why do Americans pay more money than Canadians or Europeans for the same drugs? Why do veterinarians use the same drugs, manufactured under the same standards, for America's pets, but at a fraction of the cost?"

That's just the tip of the iceberg. Dr. Felten says there are countless stories of drug companies that pay lots of money to researchers to actually promote their products. "Those people are hucksters and have egregious conflicts of interest. This practice is finally coming to light with many conspicuously bad cases that brought terrible publicity to major medical centers," he says, audibly angry.

And it's not a terribly unusual way of doing business. Dr. Felten recounted how a prestigious medical center was conducting a study on heart-rhythm problems and their surgical treatment. It researched a device that was supposed to destroy tissue that caused the heart-rhythm problem. The researchers published their findings and extolled the virtues and effectiveness of the treatment with the new device. All the buzz was promising. As it turns out, the head of the clinic where the studies were being performed and the surgeons who performed the procedure all had a vested interest in the company that created the device. In essence, they all stood to gain financially if the new procedure was a success. If they found the procedure unsuccessful, they wouldn't. For better or worse, this came to light in the media.

"How do you believe the evidence when you find out that these people stand to get huge financial rewards if the product is successful?" Dr. Felten said passionately. There's an inherent problem in how research is being done if you are directly involved in the scientific studies and also stand to gain a financial reward."

Funding is at the core of the problem, Dr. Felten explained. "Big medical schools have huge numbers of people working for them on grant money from the National Institutes of Health (NIH) and from commercial sources. In fact, most investigators are required to bring in grants to pay for their own salaries and those of technicians, post-doctorate students, and so on. But what if they're bringing money in from a commercial source? If you lose your grant money, you lose your status and perhaps your promotion and salary increases as well—perhaps even your job. Look at the pressure that puts on everyone. How many people will stick their neck out and say, 'This drug is not doing what the pharmaceutical company hopes it can achieve'? I had an experience where a pharmaceutical compound I was studying did not have the effect we had hoped. The second that data became known, the pharmaceutical company cut off the funding.

"I completely understand that a for-profit company cannot continue to fund something that does not work, but the lesson remains. If you report the data honestly and the drug does not work, the money is gone. If your job depends on the money coming in, then you're out of luck.

"There is no simple solution to such challenges, but all transactions, financial incentives, conflicts of interest, and research relationships need to become transparent and, wherever possible, managed in good faith by the institution. I do not think most researchers deliberately manipulate data or misrepresent their relationships and incentives, but there are a small number of people who scam the system for their own glory and ill-gotten gains. The majority of researchers are straightforward, ethical, conscientious people with integrity."

If Dr. Felten's commitment to "cleaning up anything not done with the utmost integrity" is as rigorous as his research and discovery of PNI, then we can feel confident that there is good leadership in important places. "The doctors at Beaumont Hospitals spend the majority of their time practicing medicine. They provide excellent care for their patients. They do research because they have questions and they want answers. They get precious little return for doing research other than the satisfaction that they have helped their patients and have contributed to our knowledge of diagnosis and treatment of disease. There's no tenure. Most are not being paid by drug companies—and if they are, they have to report it to the hospital. Beaumont Hospitals does not allow pharmaceutical reps to give anyone anything. If doctors want to meet a drug rep on their own, they can do so, but not on our campus. We do not allow free samples to be given to individual doctors, nor do we allow free trips to the Bahamas or fees for giving talks to employed physicians. That is a violation of our code of conduct.

"Many other medical schools and hospitals are putting stricter standards for conflicts of interest in place. I believe there will eventually be a national standard or code of conduct for conflict of interest rules. At this point, it takes the subpoena powers of legislators to divulge who is getting money to promote drugs. And there is still not a good way to disclose payments if the recipient chooses to out-and-out lie to their own institution, or even to the NIH, and that is not right.

"My main goal is to promote excellent research. I am relentless in pursuing honest research results that benefit our patients. There needs to be a nationwide commitment to honesty, transparency, and total integrity from the entire research community. Legitimate payments from the pharmaceutical industry to medical leaders need to be published on national sites. We need complete transparency."

Within us all there are wells of thought and dynamos of energy which are not suspected until emergencies arise.
THOMAS J. WATSON

CHAPTER 11

Dedication

*Never look down to test the ground
before taking your next step; only he
who keeps his eye fixed on the far
horizon will find the right road.*
DAG HAMMARSKJÖLD

So many qualities go into the mix of healing. You've read about many of them in this book. You've heard the stories from people who've embraced their cancer experience, released negative habits in their thinking or behavior, and healed. Literally thousands of attributes can support becoming whole and healthy on every level, but this book can't contain them all.

Like all the qualities I refer to, dedication is vital. In fact, it's fair to say that dedication—or even single-mindedness—is the center of the wheel, and the other attributes I implore you to develop are the spokes.

On the cancer journey, we're plagued with doubts about our survival.

We're traumatized by statistics. We're abused by standard treatments. We're thrown into a world where we don't recognize ourselves, and we feel useless to those we love. In many ways, life as we know it comes to an end.

But redefining life and recovering our health is possible. This book drives home that promise, and it's not possible in a single way, but in many ways. The process starts, and will be more readily achieved, if you are 100 percent dedicated to becoming well. This necessitates a blend of fully accepting what's in the present moment while maintaining a razor-sharp focus on your aspiration to be cancer free, healthy, and whole.

When we prepare for a trip, we bring out maps or Google the destination to learn more about it. As we make our plans, we figure which flights are best, which shuttles to take or which vehicle to rent, where the hotel is located, and what restaurants are nearby. These are the means for getting to the destination and making the best of it. Unless there is an unforeseen occurrence, we know we will reach our destination. We may have flashes of fear that the plane might crash or the rental car will break down, but most of us release those fears and focus on getting there *without doubt.* We are confident and easy and expect that we'll arrive.

If the trip is a vacation, the images of the destination are all the more clear and inviting. The idea of arriving is exciting; we're enthused and energized about getting there. We know the vacation will free us from our daily lives, and something about it will be liberating. It will be fun. The anticipation is palpable; we can't wait.

Even though I won't dare liken the healing journey to a fun-filled vacation, this exact brand of energy and attitude is the very best possible vehicle for carrying you through the daily hardships. Staying tuned to the destination, rather than getting bogged down in the journey, keeps the momentum in a forward direction. Having full and uncompromised confidence that *you will arrive* speaks to the cells in your body and assuages the fears.

That said, keeping your aspiration as the primary focus won't alleviate fear and pain, and it's counterproductive to pretend they aren't there. When they are, quit resisting them. Accept them. Embrace them. Know that they are part of the journey, similar to a canceled flight, uncomfortable in-flight turbulence, a noisy hotel room, or being robbed at a busy marketplace. Go through whatever grieving or anger you must, but then accept it. *Know* it will pass. Nurture yourself as deeply and lovingly as you possibly can. Pray for deliverance. Ask for help from those who love you. Go with it—and then let it go.

And always, *always* recalibrate, refocus, and dedicate your mind's eye on what you aspire to—your destination. See yourself as well. See yourself participating in life the way you want to. Feel the vibrancy you know will return. *Know* that you can be well. *Know* that you are healing. *Know* that it is possible. *Know* that you are worthy of being completely cancer free and living a full and purposeful life. *Know* that miracles happen all the time and that you are signed up for one that can absolutely come to pass. Know it as well and as certainly as you know your name, because being well is as much of who you are as the name you call yourself.

Knowing is a good place to be. Knowing is unquestionable and absolute and uplifting. We *know* we'll get to that beach and blue water under a warm and tropical sun. We *know* it's where we want to be. When we *know* things, every ounce of our physical body lines up and agrees.

I wrote this book largely because I needed to brainwash myself—or should I say, cleanse my mind of limiting thinking—so I could believe in things that others said were either impossible, unlikely, remote, or unrealistic. What I learned along the way is that they were wrong. I *know* this. I have met and spoken to many people who have either healed themselves of cancer or who know of someone who did. It happens all the time. You need to *know* this.

Professional athletes who are in it to win don't become unhinged when they fall down, miss the shot, strike out, or hit the ball into the net. They have a moment—lightning fast and intense—and then they refocus. They become totally present so they can perform their best in that moment, then the next, and then the next. By being fully present, they are able to use their skills and agility to play with the utmost excellence, hit their target, make the point, win the game. Their focus is steadfastly on achieving their goal, regardless of what they encounter along the way. They do it by being totally present.

Ironically, the most efficient way to get to your destination is to be fully present now—and to move forward with whatever comes forth.

Courage is resistance to fear, mastery of fear—not absence of fear.
MARK TWAIN

PATTY'S STORY

The power of imagination makes us infinite.
JOHN MUIR

Patty and her family run a remote resort ranch near Gunnison, Colorado, where they tend to horses, cattle, and nature-loving travelers. Like so many small-business owners, Patty's family does not have health insurance. So when she was pregnant and developed a mole on her abdomen, she avoided seeking medical advice. When the baby was two years old, however, the mole still hadn't gone away. She visited a dermatologist, who dismissed it, saying it was a maternity mole. It would cost $600 to remove it, so she opted to leave the mole alone.

As time went on, the mole turned black. In 2002, Patty sought advice from a different doctor. He took one look at it, then asked her to stay after hours so he could remove it immediately.

Patty said, "I was terrified because I knew it was bad. He cut out a cone-shaped chunk an inch in diameter. Turns out it was melanoma, stage 3." Subsequent tests revealed that a lymph node was also cancerous.

Patty was told to visit a melanoma specialist in Denver, the closest big city.

The visit cost $1,000, and she didn't know where the money would come from. Still, she knew she had to go. After removing more lymph nodes, the specialist prescribed a treatment of Interferon for a solid year.

"He told me I'd have a 70 percent chance of survival with that treatment. Of course, I followed his instructions, but the Interferon ruined me. It ruined my liver, my thyroid, my kidneys, and my teeth. My muscle mass melted away. I was really in bad shape."

While on the treatment, Patty was desperate for something to help alleviate the harsh side effects and provide her with some quality of life. A naturopathic doctor suggested that she learn and practice qigong, an ancient healing art from China. She also started taking herbs and supplements.

For about five years, things remained steady. Patty believed that with the qigong and supplements, she was faring pretty well given how much damage the Interferon had done to her body. Then in 2007, doctors found a tumor in the central-right lobe of her lung. They removed the lobe and gave her four months to live. Two months later, she lost use of her speech and the ability to use her right hand. A CT scan revealed a tumor on the left side of her brain. Doctors operated and removed the tumor, which was completely encased and had not invaded the brain.

"They wanted me to do whole-brain radiation. But one in three people go insane after that treatment. I got another opinion, and that doctor said radiation wouldn't help at all. I refused the treatment and was given two months to live. The doctor said, 'Don't bother with herbs or homeopathic remedies. You're going to die.' Then he told my daughter that if I collapsed, that meant the cancer had traveled to the brain stem. But I knew he was wrong. Since I had been doing qigong, my intuition was sharp. I just knew he was full of crap."

The same naturopath who advised Patty to practice qigong then urged her to find a doctor who practiced classical Tibetan medicine. She had nothing to lose by giving it a shot. "My daughter researched and found several different

Tibetan doctors who lived and worked in the United States. When I heard the name of one of them, this tremendous feeling of joy overwhelmed me. I said, 'That's him. That's it.'"

In Patty's first conversation with the Tibetan doctor, she asked if he could cure her. "Oh, yes. No problem," was his reply.

In that same conversation, the doctor explained specific breathing exercises called *pranayaams* that he wanted her to start performing right away.

"The MDs told me that the melanomas would pop up all over my body. I had one on my arm about two inches long and three-quarter inches wide. Within a week and a half of doing the breathing exercises, the thing was gone. Gone!"

The Tibetan doc also sent herbs, which she was instructed to take until he could visit from New York, where he lived. "He stayed with us on the ranch for three weeks. My daughter arranged for him to see patients. It was very successful. He did a lot of good for a lot of people."

She also found a world-class homeopath with a high success rate for curing cancer, and he freely gave her his recipe and instructions for treating melanoma. She then adjusted her supplement regimen to reflect what alternative cancer clinics were recommending. Finally, she began studying the healing powers of crystals and eventually became a crystal therapist.

Two years have passed since Patty was told that nothing could help her and that death was imminent. Instead of paying attention to that, she diligently performed the breathing exercises, took the herbs, practiced qigong, worked with crystals, and researched what alternative cancer centers around the world had in common, such as using pancreatic enzymes, various mushrooms, and algae. She integrated into her life a Tibetan diet that targeted her unique imbalances. She consumed Ayurvedic foods to heal her kidneys, liver, and lungs. On top of all that, she also tended to her stress level and emotional well-being.

"I took on an attitude change. I slowed down. I began to think more slowly. I studied something called 'opalescence.' That's where you remove negative emotions and transmute them into positive energy."

I asked her if, after doing all that work, she had any idea why she had gotten cancer. "Oh, yes!" she sang. "I was under a tremendous amount of anger and stress. Some people that I had loved and trusted had hurt me terribly. I had so much anger, but I've gotten rid of that. There's a direct relationship between your emotions and getting cancer. Until I did all this work, I felt that I had been unfairly treated from the time I was born. It was eating me up pretty good.

"I guess all this is leading to, I don't know, enlightenment? At least if I had time to get rid of all of my negative emotions, it would. Buddhism says that the absence of negative emotions is enlightenment."

In all the years she had worked the ranch, the idea of finding enlightenment wasn't part of Patty's mind-set, at least not before she had cancer. "I was your typical human being. I wasn't aware of this stuff at all, but the metaphysical part of my healing has been a critical piece of the whole picture. I work with angels now too. Just because we can't see everything doesn't mean it's not there. The further along I go on my journey, the more I realize that what we can't see is actually part of our reality. Changing your attitude and changing your approach to life is what you have to do to heal. The tools I've put together have helped me to make those changes."

Patty's new vigor for life has inspired her to help other people. She's currently writing a book that will feature what she learned from the Tibetan doctor, the very specific diet he created for her, her vitamin protocol, the homeopathics she's on, and how she accesses help from angels. She also plans on creating a CD and DVD that will demonstrate relaxation meditations.

Her last CT scan showed not a single tumor. "I'm done being scanned," she said confidently. "My doctor thought it was just wonderful that the cancer was gone, but he didn't want to hear about what I did."

One of the last things her doctor said was that Interferon doesn't work with melanoma. They had put her on it for a year, and suddenly he was telling her it didn't work with her particular kind of cancer. It was deeply infuriating. "But I'm being healed from all that now. My energy level is great. I leave no stone unturned, and I trust myself."

Trust is a big issue for most people. How do you go from trusting that your oncologist has your best interests at heart and is prescribing the best possible medicine to trusting your intuition?

"I don't know how to convince people of anything," Patty said. "But I'm a good case to look at. My oncologist told me that no one—*nobody*—has ever survived what I had. You have to change the way you walk, think, talk, breathe, eat. You have to meditate, get on herbs that balance you, educate yourself, read, study, and find out what appeals to you.

"I know it's hard, because when I was first diagnosed, I was scared as hell. It took a while to get the intuitive understanding of what I needed to do. It's hard to get through to people. They think they should only do what the doctors say they should do. I guess you just have to try some new things out. Know that what you did before wasn't working, or you wouldn't have gotten cancer. Disease is nature's way of telling you that your life isn't working. And healing yourself doesn't have to cost a lot of money. There are many things you can do yourself. I did."

Patty's closing words made me smile widely. "When you clean up the mess of who you are, things just get better and better. I've never been a lucky person, but now I am so lucky; things come so easily to me. Even if you don't have cancer, cleaning up your emotional life and doing the types of things I do for healing is just great. It's just a great way to live."

To learn more about Patty's upcoming book, contact her at getaway @quartercircle.net.

If you do not change direction, you may end up where you are heading.
LAO-TZU

HUIXIAN CHEN

QIGONG

I can't give you a sure-fire formula for success, but I can give you a formula for failure: try to please everybody all the time.
HERBERT BAYARD SWOPE

Huixian Chen (or Chen, as she is known) laughs easily and is playing out her seventy-six years with joy and vitality. But neither of those qualities were part of her character in years past.

"When I was a child and a young adult," she said with a Chinese accent, "I suffered a lot. I was physically very weak, and I was emotionally very troubled. Life was never stable. China was going through great distress during the anti-Japanese war. My hometown was in the south, and my whole family had to run away from the Japanese. We went through many hardships. We didn't have much to eat, and we were scared and worried all the time. In the later years, the Communist Party governed China, and I went through many different political movements. Those were hard for people too. We had to survive politically, be among the progressive people, or be left behind. We had to work hard and speak positively. We were always afraid that we might be exposed, or that someone might make rumors about us and then we'd be punished. This kind of political worry was very intense.

"I was very depressed. I married, but was not happy in my marriage. All these emotional things accumulated in me, and I didn't feel well at all. In 1983, while I was still living in Beijing, I was finally diagnosed with stage 4 breast cancer. They operated on me and took out nineteen lymph nodes. All of them were full of cancer. According to my doctor, my entire body was invaded by cancer; my whole lymph system was cancer ridden."

After a mastectomy, the doctors told Chen to try chemo, but they cautioned that it would only give her about a 25 percent chance of survival. "I was hospitalized for a month so that they could administer the chemo. It was very strong back then, and my body couldn't stand it. I was so weak I couldn't eat or even drink water. Whatever I took into my mouth, I would throw up. I thought I could not go on.

"I took some Chinese herbs, which made it possible for me to eat a little, but I couldn't sleep. For many years before I had cancer, I struggled with insomnia. I had to take sleeping pills every night, but they would only work for two, three, or four hours. And then I would get up to work. I developed a terrible habit with that.

"During the time of radiation treatment, I couldn't sleep at all. I was very depressed. I thought I was going to die. I was forty-nine years old and had two children. One was older and in college, but the other was only nine. I worried about them. I thought that if I died, they would suffer. I was very sad, and I cried a lot."

The radiation wasn't working, but the universe was. While in the waiting room for a radiation treatment, Chen started conversing with another patient. He inquired about her situation, and she told him that she was going to die since the cancer was everywhere in her body. "He listened to my story very patiently and then said, 'Oh, don't worry. Let me tell you my story, then you'll have confidence.'"

The stranger explained to Chen that he had been diagnosed with late-stage lung cancer. "My two lungs were filled with big and small cancers," he said. "The doctors couldn't do anything to help me. I was told to go home. But I didn't want to give up, so I went out from the small town where I lived to Beijing, looking for hope. The doctors here said there was nothing they could do and sent me home.

"One day I passed a park where people were doing exercises. It was new to me. I went to the group and asked what they were doing. They told me they were all cancer patients and were practicing qigong. I asked them what it was, and they said understanding it didn't matter. They told me just to join them."

The man practiced qigong with the group for a month and felt much better. He decided to return to the doctor and get checked, but the doctor assured him there was no point; the man's condition was terminal. The man pushed the doctor to run some tests, and he finally relented. After drawing blood and taking scans and X-rays, the doctor was surprised and said, "There is only one cancer left. Where have all those other cancers gone?" After that, the doctor said the man could undergo radiation for the last remaining tumor.

"And that is where we met," Chen said, "in the waiting room for radiation. He encouraged me to go to the cancer-qigong group. I figured if there were any way I could help myself, I would. He was very kind. He bought me a monthly pass to the park so that I could go. I began by learning something called soaring crane qigong. At the beginning, it was hard to do the movements because the operation I'd had made it difficult to lift my right arm. I tried my best even though I wasn't up to the standard.

"Within three weeks, I felt a difference in my life. I could sleep much better. I could eat more. I felt happier, less depressed. Day by day, I was feeling better. After one month of doing qigong every day, I felt that I was myself again, and I was so happy. I started talking about qigong to everyone I met."

After her doctor conducted the usual tests, he determined that Chen was completely cancer free. Even though the doctor was trained in Western medicine, he was soon promoting qigong for his other cancer patients.

Around that same time, Chen learned about the power behind the healing energy of qigong. "I went to a shop to buy something for my children. The shop was very crowded, and I accidentally touched the button of a woman's overcoat. She screamed and said, 'What did you do to me?' I told her I did nothing. She said, 'You put a knife into my body!' I promised her that I did not. Other people in the store thought I had done something, too. I looked down at my own fingers and said aloud, 'What's that? Electricity?' The woman was so frightened she ran away.

"I went back to the park and told my teacher what had happened. He told me not to worry because the energy the woman had felt was *qi,* or life force. He told me that I had inadvertently put some of my qi into the woman, and it scared her. He told me that people can emit the energy, but that I should keep it to myself for my own healing because he didn't think I was completely healthy yet. He told me that someday, when I was really good at qigong, I could use it to help heal other people."

Chen explained that the healing property of qigong isn't just a gift that she was given; it's possible for anyone and everyone to access.

"Qi is bioenergy. Everyone has it by nature; everyone is born with it. Qi is the life force, and without it, you could not live. It's with you as soon as you are born. Some people use it to heal others, but instead of depending on other people's qi, it's best to cultivate it yourself."

After she was healed, Chen realized that her mission was to expose as many people as possible to qigong. Even though she had spent years teaching English at the University of International Business and Economics in Beijing, her passion for qigong inspired her to practice until she was qualified to teach. In 1986, she went to Arizona as an exchange scholar, where she taught Chinese business language to Americans. By then, she had mastered her qigong techniques and in her spare time taught qigong classes to curious Americans. She traveled back and forth between China and America for years, all the while teaching this ancient healing art.

When Chen retired from the university in Beijing, she decided to teach qigong full time. Fortuitously, in 1993, she moved to Portland, Oregon, where she was invited to teach qigong at the Oregon College of Oriental Medicine.

"I was sixty years old when I started my new career. Over the years I have traveled all over Canada, Europe, and the United States, and I've certified more than four hundred teachers in qigong. That's on top of the tens of thousands of students who have taken my classes."

Chen has worked with many students who've had cancer and are now completely healthy. Clearly, qigong is powerful medicine, but I was curious as to whether Chen thought emotional issues, in part, caused cancer. "Most of the time, cancer is related to emotional disease. Most of the people I've worked with who've had cancer also had emotional problems. Emotions decide the health condition. It doesn't necessarily have to be cancer, but if something goes wrong emotionally, it will affect the body right away.

"I look at my own life. My childhood years were very, very difficult. I used to be so depressed that I thought everyone around me was laughing at me and looking down upon me. If people were talking in low voices, I thought they were gossiping about me. I was so suspicious. Also in my marriage I was very unhappy, but how could I express it? The only way was to quarrel and argue, but still that didn't solve the problem. I felt always a feeling of suffocation in the chest—and that's where I got cancer.

"When I first got cancer, I didn't realize that it was because of emotions. As I practiced qigong, it changed my outlook. I started seeing things in a different way. Practicing qigong opens our channels, our minds, and our acupoints so we can communicate with the universe. I believe there are a lot of positive things in the universe—positive inspiration, positive feelings. As soon as I got in touch with qi, the universe, I began to open up. I became as loving, forgiving, and generous as the universe, so naturally the feeling of suffocation in my chest went away. It's very interesting. Whenever I didn't feel well, I did qigong and immediately I felt OK.

"Qigong is the way I healed both physically and emotionally. Now if someone is rude to me, I don't get angry at all. I see no fault in anybody. I just let go. Now life is so easy."

The mystery of why qigong heals cancer—and a host of other diseases—led me to ask Chen, in the simplest of terms, to explain what qigong is. Her reply was elegant: "Qigong is a traditional Chinese technique that's been used for five thousand years to teach people how to get in touch with the source of life."

I didn't feel the need to ask Chen about her diet and how it may have played a role in her healing. Clearly, her practice of qigong changed both her state of mind and the health of her cells. I did ask if she wanted to offer anything else about healing from cancer.

"Open your mind to accept all kinds of possibilities for healing. Consciousness is so important," she answered.

Chen now lives in California and devotes her time to teaching advanced classes. Qigong classes are offered all over the United States. To learn more about the healing properties and possibilities, visit Chen's website at wis domandpeace.com.

The only tyrant I accept in this world is the still voice within.
MAHATMA GANDHI

TULLIO SIMONCINI, MD

Author of *Cancer Is a Fungus: A Revolution in Tumor Therapy*

It is only by following your deepest instinct that you can lead a rich life.
KATHARINE BUTLER HATHAWAY

"The soul and the body are not two separate and noncommunicating domains, but two manifestations of the same being and equally responsible for the health of an individual. It is the entire individual who must be considered, both in his vital dynamics and from a psychological and even spiritual perspective, even if these can't be measured.

"It is in this area that the failure of medicine is most glaring.... This happens especially in the area of oncology, where a deep state of confusion and resignation is felt the most.

"Genetics, the battle horse of modern oncology, is about to give up the ghost, together with its endless explanations based on enzymatic and receptor processes. Actually, it has already failed—it's just that no one can think of anything else that can take its place. The consequence of the oncological establishment's inability to admit the failure of this line of research, which is at this point scientifically indefensible, is the continuous waste of a great quantity of economic, scientific, and human resources."[1]

Such is the heartfelt and controversial point of view written in the introduction of Dr. Tullio Simoncini's book *Cancer Is a Fungus: A Revolution in Tumor Therapy.*

***

My overseas telephone conversation with Dr. Simoncini echoed his battle cry that researchers in the US or European countries have no freedom to test new ways of treating cancer. The drug companies alone, he says, dictate what kind of research is permitted. Dr. Simoncini lives in Italy, where the cancer culture is apparently under the same pharmaceutical stranglehold as in the US.

"The people who have the ability to research new modes for cancer treatment are protecting the institutions with power, who want to keep things the way they are," he claimed in a heavy Italian accent. "Chemo is just a mess. It gets you sicker. But the power and politics behind medicine make it very hard for doctors to even try new and different treatments. They are afraid to try because it goes against those who hold the power."

Dr. Simoncini knows firsthand what the power that propels the medical world can do to disrupt the practice of innovative doctors and researchers. Thirty years ago, while working as an internist, Dr. Simoncini was successfully treating psoriasis, a skin disorder, with iodine. It became clear to him that psoriasis was actually a fungus that resulted in infection. Expanding this line of thinking, Dr. Simoncini considered that if infection was behind the manifestation of psoriasis, couldn't infection also be the reason for the creation of tumors?

While working in a pediatric ward, Dr. Simoncini observed how children with thrush (candida on the tongue) responded well to sodium bicarbonate (baking soda) as a treatment. He conjectured that since candida is a fungus, it could also be the result of an underlying infection. If so, he surmised that candida could possibly cause tumors. He decided to test his theory to see if sodium bicarbonate would dissolve tumors.

His first case was in the late 1970s. A mother had taken her eleven-year-old boy to the university where Simoncini worked. The child had been in a coma for fifteen days due to a metastasis of lymphoma in his brain. Dr. Simoncini began sodium bicarbonate infusions at 11:30 in the morning, the same day the boy entered the hospital ward. By that evening, the boy woke up and was able to go to the restroom by himself.

Another significant case that Dr. Simoncini remembers took place in 1983. The patient had lung cancer. After nine months of receiving intravenous sodium bicarbonate for six out of seven days per week, every week, the man was completely cancer free.

Naturally, Dr. Simoncini was thrilled with the results. Much to his dismay, however, his colleagues at the university refused to cooperate with him to administer the protocol on other patients. "The medical community that I thought would applaud such positive results turned against me," he said. "Other doctors weren't ready for this. I was persecuted, ostracized, and disbarred. Even though I could no longer practice medicine with patients, I didn't stop my work. I consulted. I now speak about it scientifically. I can advise people. I have collaborators in Italy, Switzerland, and Spain." Some of his collaborators are surgeons, doctors, and other medical professionals who had cancer themselves and, after listening to his advice, are now tumor free.

He also advises patients to treat themselves. "People call me from all over the world—America, the UK, Columbia, South Africa, Croatia, Australia, Mexico—everywhere. Doctors call me because they want my scientific point of view."

The science comes down to this: tumors, according to Dr. Simoncini, are candida, a fungal infection. "The simple application of sodium bicarbonate can dissolve the tumor. It's no more complicated than that."

Dr. Simoncini explains that the fungal infection is on the outside of the cell rather than on the inside. He believes washing the cell of the fungus is all that's necessary to shrink the tumor. "Tumors have nothing to do with genes, enzymes, or receptors," he continues. "Cancer is not an intercellular disorder. It is purely a fungal infection on the outside of the cell."

According to Dr. Simoncini, thousands of patients around the world with every imaginable kind of cancer have successfully become tumor free after applying his protocol. Since baking soda is available everywhere, and since it is not a toxic substance, some patients can treat themselves if they get appropriate advice. However, very few doctors openly practice this treatment. Self-treatment may be partly why the medical world has rejected his work. Dr. Simoncini believes it's too simple, too accessible, and too affordable to support the greed behind the cancer industry.

Even with all his successes, however, sodium bicarbonate doesn't work for every type of cancer. Those without an identifiable target, or whose tumors are not accessible, do not respond. Most others do—and patients can see results sometimes within twenty-four hours.

"People who have not been treated with chemotherapy or radiation respond much better to this treatment because they still have a reserve of energy. Those who have been destroyed by oncology have a harder time, and then there are those who come to me when it's too late."

Medications widely used to treat blood pressure, diabetes, and heart disease, according to Dr. Simoncini, weaken the organs and favor fungal invasion. "This is one of the most important things to know about what causes cancer. When organs are weak, the fungus, candida, takes over, and cancer is present."

The passion that Dr. Simoncini expresses for his successes is only matched by his frustration about the close-minded nature of the cancer industry. When asked what he thinks it will take to change the culture, Dr. Simoncini looks to the Chinese. "They do not care about the power that Western medicine holds. They don't want to accept the power of Western medicine. They are doing alternative research because they want to manage things differently. They will ultimately destroy the system that's in place right now. When people start to experience their ways of healing cancer, we will have the end of power in this medical area. Right now in the Western countries, there is no freedom to practice alternative treatments for cancer. No freedom."

On the brighter side, Dr. Simoncini claims he has between 70 and 80 percent success rates when patients are not terminal or with metastasis.

I asked him how the mind contributes to the cure. He's a credentialed philosopher, but his perspective was straightforward and down-to-earth. "If you want to get well, you have to learn to control your energy. You have to manage your own energy intellectually, mentally, spiritually, and physically. Most people don't manage it well because it's difficult. It's an ethical issue, a moral issue. You have to sacrifice something to do it, such as diet. You can't eat just for pleasure. You can't drink too much or eat too many sweets or too much pork. I like to eat everything, but I have to monitor everything I do. I like to have a social life, but I can't do parties all the time. I have to control my energy if I want to reach a bigger goal. Same with consumption. I cannot buy three houses or cars that I cannot pay for. I cannot work enough to buy them.

"These choices are important. They contribute to your wellness. During the day, you have many opportunities to face many choices. You must balance the spiritual in the middle of your day. You can do whatever you want, but you need to know when to do it. If you balance these things, you drop off the heavy weights in your soul and spirit. You can be more free."

Dr. Simoncini believes that emotional weight contributes to severe illness and must be handled before it turns into a physical manifestation. Otherwise, it compounds the problem. "We must be moral and forgive the sins of other people."

Even so, he believes that emotional and physical issues must be addressed independently of one another. "Sometimes alternative doctors make this mistake. They treat the emotional illness to heal the physical problem, but that rarely heals the body. It is important to eliminate the physical problem because it may be too late to manage the emotional issue."

Dr. Simoncini, who is a musician and believes in the power of beauty, suggests also that people with cancer surround themselves with what they love. "Music is the sound of the vibrations of life. The greatest vibration is when you can give love to somebody and have love come back because the vibrations hit you totally, and you can multiply them with the vibrations of all that is. In my opinion, the Christian message has to be followed in its essence."

Unfortunately, it's not easy to find practitioners who can administer Dr. Simoncini's sodium bicarbonate treatments. Most people fly to Rome and work with him firsthand. His book explains the science behind his discoveries, specific types of treatments, and which cancers respond most favorably.

Scientific Support for Sodium Bicarbonate Treatment

Dr. Simoncini's use of sodium bicarbonate to successfully reduce or eliminate cancerous tumors might now be explained scientifically. A study was collaboratively conducted by researchers at the Arizona Cancer Center at the University of Arizona at Tucson, Wayne State University in Detroit, and the H. Lee Moffit Cancer Center and Research Institute in Tampa, Florida. The paper resulting from that study is entitled, "Bicarbonate Increases Tumor pH and Inhibits Spontaneous Metastases."[2] For those who can decipher scientific papers, you can get a reprint of it by contacting Robert Gillies, H. Lee Moffitt Cancer Center, SRB-2, 12302 Magnolia Drive, Tampa, FL 33612. Phone: 813-725-8355; Fax: 813-979-7265; E-mail: Robert.Gillies@moffitt.org. If you're not able to read scientific studies, e-mail Dr. Simoncini and ask him what it means. He will likely be happy to tell you.

To learn more about Dr. Simoncini, go to cancerfungus.com or e-mail him at t.simoncini@alice.it.

You desire to know the art of living, my friend?
It is contained in one phrase: make use of suffering.
HENRI FREDERIC AMIEL

CHAPTER 12

Trust

Your fulfillment lies not in obtaining the objects of your desire, but in the unfoldment of your soul qualities in making the effort to succeed in worthwhile endeavors.
PARAMAHANSA YOGANANDA

It's easy to say, "OK, I'll trust this process once I'm healed." The twist, however, is that trusting the process *before* there's evidence of healing is a necessary component of the healing process.

Trusting that your cancer experience is one that can awaken you to great love, beauty, power, and knowledge feels like risky business. But it's only risky if expectations cage you in, so you settle for a specific end-point for that experience. Trust is giving yourself to *what is* and believing that *what is* cannot shake who you really are. But that means you have to trust that who you really are is bigger than the cancer—whether you become cancer free or not.

Being able to trust is huge. It's been the most elusive of all qualities for me to harness. In moments throughout my cancer experience, I've been so tightly gripped by fear—and disconnected from trust—that I have temporarily lost my senses.

I'm beginning to understand that fear is something that I will probably live with forever. But my relationship with fear is changing. Rather than having it grip me, I have learned how to hold it. Rather than being in the bowels of it, I am now able to be on the outside of it. I have come to know it—even empathize with it—and I now understand that it is very often a signal that I am simply not trusting.

One sleepless night when I was fighting the fear that was creeping up my spine, I finally gave up resistance and gave myself to it. I wanted to follow it to the source. I couldn't understand why I still had such intense bouts of fear, and decided that I had nothing to lose by simply getting to know it.

What I discovered is something that I believe may live within most of us. I went to a place so hidden and dark that I perceived it as a cavern beneath the ocean floor of my subconscious mind. It was primordial and ancient. It felt like a surreptitious gathering place for all judgment, guilt, and self-loathing that I had collected throughout all of my incarnations. It is where unhealed wounds fester and create the breeding ground for fear.

When I found it, I instantly had empathy for the fear. I realized that the fear was not out to destroy me; rather, it was simply a product of what others called my shadow self. It's a mythical place that the rational mind can't figure out. The fear speaks of that place. It is a messenger.

The only thing I know to do with this cavern is to offer it love and to trust that by doing so it will somehow be transformed.

In his book *Radical Forgiveness,* Colin Tipping refers to this place of fear.[1] He offers simple exercises that can release subconscious habits borne of the separation that is harbored there.

His tools are easy to use and provide an accessible way to relieve the trauma that our shadow self creates. But there is a purpose for this shadow, too. By going there and shedding light upon it, we can finally trust that even fear is an important part of who we are.

Trust is the sister of peace; it has no need or desire to fight or to blame. It dwells in a milieu of calm and quiet and knows that no matter what happens, we are here to evolve.

Trust is an invisible insulation that protects us from the storms of life, enabling us to look out at them with an unbending sense of well-being.

Trust is when we believe that, regardless of the outcome we're after, our journey is right. It is in sync with a divine purpose, and it knows that we are not alone in our efforts to prevail. Trust is the acceptance of all that is, and being calm in the midst of uncertainty.

We are not what we know but what we are willing to learn.
MARY CATHERINE BATESON

LINDA'S STORY

*How we spend our days is, of course,
how we spend our lives.*
ANNIE DILLARD

"At some point, you just have to say, 'I created this. I trust that I have it for some reason, so now I'll make the best of it.'"

According to fifty-nine-year-old Linda, turning challenges into something positive isn't so difficult when you believe that the root of whatever happens in life is your divine path unfolding and inviting you to evolve. I wholeheartedly agree with that. Still, after hearing her story, it took me a few head shakes, deep breaths, and contemplative moments to grasp exactly how she has come to such a deep, unflappable trust in a life crowded with so much hardship.

"It came over time," she said, admitting that she hadn't possessed her deep-seated trust when she'd been diagnosed with a severe case of rheumatoid arthritis. "I felt totally victimized," she reported with a quiet calm that hummed throughout our conversation. "I was a twenty-year-old woman in an eighty-year-old body. The pain would go away when I was pregnant or nursing, but then it would come back ferociously. I had hand surgeries; I took drugs; I did it all. But after my second child, it was so bad I couldn't lift the baby, and I had to hire someone to help."

Eventually, Linda decided to begin taking responsibility for her condition. She started to exercise and that felt good. Then she took up swimming and felt even better.

"I determined that part of how I would heal was by getting outside of myself, so I started to raise money to build a pool at the hospital, a warm pool. We ran articles in the paper, and I got thousands of responses from people with different types of diseases, all of which would respond well to a warm pool. The political forces between two medical facilities started bickering about who would build it, but I kept focusing on what would be healing for as many people as possible."

Her dedication was strong, and two years after she first conceived of the idea, the pool was built. Now, three decades later, the pool continues to serve tens of thousands of people at a well-respected regional hospital.

Linda's attitude about the success of the project remains modest. "I didn't do it for recognition. It was really for my own development. I did it so that I could learn what I needed to learn about myself."

Around the time the pool was being constructed, she also began assembling a platform for her spiritual understanding. Learning about herself became a central theme. She came to this in part when she sought an energetic or nonphysical explanation of why she had the arthritis. According to the work of Louise Hay (louisehay.com), rheumatoid arthritis represents a spiritual receding from the life force, a lack of engagement in this life, and a lack of flexibility in character.

"I began looking at that," she said. "I was a really strong personality that believed it was my way or the highway. I believed I was right and everyone else was wrong." Hay's interpretation of the disease opened her to change, and she was soon able to see that what was right for her wasn't necessarily right for everyone else. This newfound insight was tested in the extreme throughout the coming years.

By the time Linda's son, Seth, was seven years old, he had already been through the ringer. At six months of age, he had contracted encephalitis. Doctors told Linda and her husband, John, that the infection had destroyed half of Seth's brain and that they should place him in an institution. But Seth's parents refused, and within an appropriate time frame, he was walking and talking. Doctors then urged them to put Seth in a school for children with developmental disabilities. Again, Linda and John said no, wanting instead for their son to be around other kids who could demonstrate to Seth what his greatest potential could be.

But before he was to enroll in first grade, Seth needed to have surgery to lengthen the heel cord in his leg, a necessary procedure to mitigate complications from the encephalitis. At the same time, doctors would repair a hernia—quite an operation for such a little boy.

Things went well until three weeks after the surgery. Linda recounts the story between a string of long pauses: "One night, he woke up screaming. They did tests for weeks, but nothing showed up. They finally did a CT scan and found lymphoma everywhere. He was airlifted to a children's hospital where an alert team stayed with him around the clock. One of his kidneys had stopped functioning, and the other was starting to fail. The chemo they ran through him was so hard on him, they didn't know if he would make it. The cancer doubled every twenty-four hours."

Linda's voice shook. "At one point, I called a psychic I had seen before all this happened. She had told me that Seth would grow up to be six foot three. I let her know what was going on. She said she didn't know what would happen, but there was so much light pouring into him from the many people praying for him, and that if anyone could make it, Seth could."

One month after he'd been airlifted to the hospital, all of his organs were back to normal. Linda believes the combination of chemo and prayers saved her son.

Making it through that tenuous month didn't guarantee that he'd grow up to be six foot three. In fact, doctors gave Seth just a 50 percent chance of survival. He underwent chemotherapy every two weeks for the next two years, and during that time, he had eighteen spinal taps.

This is when Linda really amped up her spiritual practice. "I wanted him to live, and I was doing everything I could to make him want to live. Then I realized that I was imposing onto him my desire that he live. Someone I worked with helped me to see that. It was the whole arthritis thing—imposing my will on him.

"After many tears, I gained a new understanding. I had to give him the freedom to be here or to go. I finally became OK if he wanted to go. I felt that I had to give him that. It was the very best way I could support him."

As Linda took a moment to breathe, I wondered what parent wouldn't impose their desire on a child in those circumstances. I know I would. She went on: "The next day he was so happy. He was playing the song 'New Attitude' and put his underwear on his head. He said, 'I've graduated, and it's time for you to graduate, too!' Then he put the underwear on my head, and we danced.

"I believe you come to this life to do certain work. You learn things about yourself, and ultimately you help heal the planet when you do work on yourself."

Linda believes there is nothing random about what happens to us. "When Seth was four years old," she elaborated, "we were sitting in the hot tub, looking at the moon. He told me that once upon a time he and his older brother were sitting on the moon, watching John and me cook dinner. Seth looked at his brother and said, 'We can be happy there. We can go there.'

"That was the story of how he chose John and me as his parents. You choose everything. You pick a path and declare that there are certain things you want to learn, and you decide how you'll bring healing to yourself and the planet.

"I set off to have arthritis so that I would expand and learn and help to heal the planet. That was my choice in life, just as my sons knew that by choosing us, they'd have a secure place to do their work."

At seven years old, Seth was doing great. Not long after surgery, and while still doing the chemo, he was ready for the first grade. He had always dreamed of riding a school bus, and on the first day of school, he insisted on walking to the bus stop. For most kids, that would be no big deal, but the cast from the surgery had only recently been removed. Plus, he was small in stature and weak from the chemo. Still, he was determined to walk by himself and ride the bus. John and Linda agreed that he could, but secretly followed him, hiding behind bushes so he couldn't spot them.

Seth arrived at the bus stop by himself without incident, but was unable to make it up the steps of the bus. It didn't phase him. With the bus driver's help, Seth found himself in the bus, ready to take on his first day of school. His parents were elated, and their son had realized his dream.

Years passed without incident, but then something else came into play. When her boys were in high school and she was forty-two, Linda was diagnosed with breast cancer.

"That's when the real lessons of trust came," she proclaimed, her cadence in full swing again. "I did chemo and radiation, but the cancer came right back. I looked at the bigger picture and came to understand that the cancer had to do with me taking on the role of *mother of the world.* I mothered not only everybody in my family, but everyone else too!

"I chose to have a double mastectomy, and after that, I realized that we all have our own path. I didn't need to take care of anyone else anymore, except myself. I began to trust that everything—*everything*—is our own creation so that we can learn about ourselves and heal."

Six years after her bout with breast cancer, Linda's arthritis flared up badly.

"I was trusting the path by then and no longer asked myself why I couldn't heal it. I had to stop asking and instead trust that I would have it as long as I needed to. I was no longer a victim. I accepted that I had created it all. I came here to do this. It's my path, and I have to trust it, whatever happens.

"To question your path is futile. You just have to go with it. It all comes down to trust, creation, and healing, both of yourself and of the planet, and that means you understand oneness. So, for instance, when I understood that my cancer had to do with overmothering, I put that thought form out into the world so that everyone could have access to it. It's like the collective unconscious. When you learn about yourself, ultimately the knowledge is there for everyone."

Linda has been cancer free for eighteen years, and no longer experiences pain from the rheumatoid arthritis. She continues to practice her spiritual beliefs by diligently attending to both her physical and nonphysical bodies. "If you saw X-rays of my feet, you'd be amazed that I can walk at all.

I have weak, loose joints, and can't be on my feet for long. I take small doses of a cancer drug and medication for the arthritis. I believe I healed myself, but I'm not getting off the pills to test it."

In the mix of how our paths unfold, Linda agrees that destructive subconscious thoughts definitely need to be released. She spent years using muscle testing as a way to free herself of limiting beliefs. But she doesn't buy into the notion of karma or past lives. "It's all now. Life is all now. If you think you have something leftover from another life, it's such a guilt thing. It's not empowering. The whole point is to become empowered. We are all master creators with choices.

"You have the ability to heal yourself. That's a choice you make, but it may not be the path that the bigger part of you—the divine part—makes. When you limit yourself to what you want, you might miss the bigger story of creation. If I woke up tomorrow racked with pain from the arthritis, I wouldn't beat myself up. I wouldn't be happy, but I would trust that I created it. I would want to be pain free, but if I weren't, I would accept it.

"Outcomes don't matter. All that matters is what we learn about ourselves. Whether I live or die, I will heal. Either I heal myself, or I will die and then I will heal. If my path is to die, then the people around me will learn about themselves, which will be my gift to them.

"In life's journey, there are choices in every moment. My choice was to live. It was intertwined with trusting that my spiritual path would actually determine whether I would live or die. If I had died, it would have been my divine self making that choice. Again, that's where trust comes in. There's a bigger picture going on. By second-guessing the bigger picture, you lose touch with your divine nature and what you can learn about yourself."

At the time of our interview, Seth was thirty-one years of age and six foot three. He recently earned a master's degree in journalism and has been accepted into a program for a second master's, this time in psychology.

Linda and John have been married since 1971. Their partnership is shared both personally and through a business they have created. They travel often and delight in whatever shows up on any given day, believing with profound and exemplary trust that they're creating it all. They carry it out with joy, with the promise to heal themselves, and they offer the gift of well-being and wholeness to all who will embrace it.

Let a joy keep you.
Reach out your hands
And take it when it runs by.
CARL SANDBURG

JEREMY GEFFEN, MD, FACP

Multidimensional Beings
Author of *The Journey Through Cancer: Healing and Transforming the Whole Person*

To realize one's nature perfectly—that is what each of us is here for.
OSCAR WILDE

"I see humans as multidimensional beings. We each have a physical body, a mind, a heart, and a spiritual dimension. We are all also deeply interconnected to each other, to nature, and to the entire cosmos in ways that transcend our usual experience of feeling separate and that defy conventional understanding. If medicine and healing are to be as complete as possible, we must honor and care for *all* these dimensions and all these interconnections, with equal skill and integrity, including the parts that are buried deep within."

I didn't hear this from a monk, although Jeremy Geffen, when he was living in an ashram as a young man, seriously contemplated becoming one. Instead, he became a highly trained, board-certified, medical oncologist. A summa cum laude graduate of Columbia University, he received his MD with honors from New York University School of Medicine, and he is now a fellow of the American College of Physicians.

So how did Dr. Geffen go from studying great spiritual and healing traditions and practicing yoga and meditation for hours every day to the scientific and technological field of modern oncology with all its bells and whistles?

"I was chosen for this path. There's no doubt about it," he told me from his office in Boulder, Colorado. "After I'd spent four years at the ashram, a voice in my heart called me to become a physician. It wouldn't leave me alone. So after a tender farewell, I left to pursue a career in medicine."

Geffen chose oncology within his first week at medical school. During a series of lectures about various specialties, he "lit up inside" when the oncologist came to the podium and spoke about caring for people with cancer.

"I realized that people with cancer are living on the edge of two worlds. They are dealing with complex medical issues, and they need the best that modern science and technology have to offer. But they are also quite often staring into the abyss of the unknown, grappling with some of life's greatest challenges and uncertainties. So they need love, wisdom, and compassionate guidance as well.

"Cancer often challenges the mind, heart, and spirit as deeply as—if not more deeply than—the physical body. The question then is, what is the most conscious, empowered, enlightened, and effective way to respond?"

That question fueled him through four years of medical school, a three-year residency in internal medicine at the University of California at San Diego, and three more years of fellowship training in hematology and oncology at the University of California at San Francisco. What ensued was that Dr. Geffen became a pioneer in the emerging fields of integrative medicine and oncology.

While his scientific mind was fully engaged, his spiritual heart continued to grow. He learned everything he could from various teachers in India, Nepal, China, and Tibet, and on a Native American reservation. Ultimately, what shaped his life and practice was a deep desire to know how to "honor and care for every single dimension of human beings, and not just treat the body as though it were simply a machine."

It seems few MDs maintain such high expectations of themselves and their patients. But Dr. Geffen isn't your typical oncologist. In our conversation, he expressed deep empathy for his patients and families because of his own life experience. In 1985, while he was a senior in medical school, his father died of stomach cancer. This made him painfully aware of the limitations of both allopathic and alternative medicine, the lack of emotional and spiritual support available to patients, and the humiliating and disempowering feelings that so many cancer patients experience. Ultimately, it propelled him to create something better, and it shaped how he both lives and works.

"My father died less than four months after his diagnosis. Being in that crucible with him was devastating. My mind and heart were blown open when I directly experienced what people often go through in facing the challenges of cancer and death.

"During my father's illness, we were surrounded by brilliant oncologists who understood the biology and genetics of cancer and who had access to all the latest technologies of modern medicine. But by and large, they were uninformed about any potential benefits of complementary or alternative therapies, or the power and gifts of many of the world's other healing traditions. They were also unable to deal with the overwhelming impact of cancer on my father's mind, heart, and spirit, and on our family.

"On my father's journey through cancer, we also met with many wonderful complementary and alternative practitioners. They were good and caring people, but with all due respect, most knew very little about the biology and genetics of cancer, let alone the ins and outs of modern, conventional cancer treatments. Nor were they equipped to adequately care for people who were as sick as my father."

Dr. Geffen's frustration mounted. He knew from his travels and years in the ashram that there were many things that could help, but no one was offering or even considering them. "I couldn't stop asking myself, 'How can all of the great healing modalities of the world be woven together into a tapestry that skillfully and effectively addresses the needs and concerns of the whole person?'

"After my father died, I decided to become the kind of oncologist that I wished had been there for my dad, someone who could blend the world's many healing traditions together with conventional Western medicine in a safe and meaningful way. I wanted to be a doctor who could peer as deeply into a patient's heart and soul as I could into their CT scans, blood-test results, or pathology reports.

"I became possessed by a singular question: what does it take for a human being to heal and transform at the deepest levels of the body, mind, heart, and spirit in the face of cancer?

"I was intensely motivated to find answers. I vowed to build a cancer center and create a model of care that would integrate the best of the world's healing traditions and show how to honor and care for every dimension of human beings within the context of modern medicine. I realized that this is what I was born to do."

And so, in 1994, he founded the Geffen Cancer Center and Research Institute in Vero Beach, Florida, which he directed until 2003. It was among the first cancer centers in the United States explicitly designed to be a working model for treating the whole person, multidimensionally, with integrative cancer care.

Soon after opening the center, he recognized that all the needs, questions, and concerns of patients and their loved ones fell elegantly into seven fundamental domains of inquiry and exploration. It wasn't long before he organized what he calls the Seven Levels of Healing into a formal program, which, along with state-of-the-art conventional treatments and a wide array of complementary therapies, became the basis of the care he and his staff provided to thousands of patients and loved ones over the next ten years.

Dr. Geffen explained, "Understanding these levels helps people navigate all dimensions of the cancer journey with skill, awareness, and depth and transforms the experience at every step along the way. These levels are universal and apply to any healing journey, whether related to cancer, other illness, or life itself."

In 2000, he published the first edition of his book *The Journey Through Cancer: Healing and Transforming the Whole Person,* which describes the Seven Levels of Healing and his revolutionary approach to whole person care.[2] Briefly, the Seven Levels are as follows:

- **Level 1**—Education and Information: provides basic knowledge and information about modern cancer diagnosis and treatment.

- **Level 2**—Connection with Others: focuses on the need for and benefits of a strong support network on the journey through cancer.

- **Level 3**—The Body as Garden: explores the safe and effective use of complementary therapies, and invites patients and family members to regard the body as a sacred and wondrously complex garden rather than just a machine.

- **Level 4**—Emotional Healing: Helps patients and families deal effectively with the emotional issues and challenges often encountered when dealing with cancer.
- **Level 5**—The Nature of Mind: explores how our thoughts and beliefs—and the meanings we give to events—influence every aspect of our experience on the journey through cancer, and, indeed, life itself.
- **Level 6**—Life Assessment: helps patients and family members to discover the deepest meaning and purpose of their lives and their most important goals.
- **Level 7**—The Nature of Spirit: connects patients and loved ones to the profoundly healing spiritual dimension of life that we all share.

In 2003, Dr. Geffen closed the Geffen Cancer Center and relocated to Boulder to work full time to bring the Seven Levels of Healing to a wider audience and to advance an integrative, multidimensional, whole-person approach to cancer care. His company, Geffen Visions International, is dedicated to this mission. The program is now being offered to patients, loved ones, and health professionals at a growing number of cancer centers throughout the United States. In 2006, he published a fully updated second edition of *The Journey Through Cancer.*

Given his holistic approach, I figured Dr. Geffen would appreciate and even advocate alternative therapies. Generally speaking, however, he doesn't. He makes a distinction between alternative and complementary therapies, defining alternative therapies as those that are scientifically unproven, have unknown or potentially adverse interactions with conventional treatments, and are sometimes used instead of conventional treatment.

Complementary therapies refer to a wide array of modalities: diet and nutritional support, yoga, massage, acupuncture, mind-body interventions, and energy therapies. These may or may not be scientifically proven, but are increasingly found to be safe and helpful when used in conjunction with conventional care.

Although Dr. Geffen acknowledges that some alternative therapies may anecdotally appear to be effective, he says that based on his understanding of medicine and oncology, and his personal experience with cancer patients, he believes that they are unreliable and largely ineffective. He believes they rarely address the deeper dimensions of what people with cancer are encountering in their minds, hearts, and spirits, as well as their physical bodies.

At the same time, as loyal as Geffen is to his profession, he also concedes that surgery, chemotherapy, and radiation are not the holy grail either. "To be honest, mainstream cancer therapies cannot usually cure cancer once it has metastasized. At the same time, we now have many powerful diagnostic tools, drugs, surgical techniques, and radiation technologies that can be very helpful and even extend survival. But these technologies and the benefits they bring often come at a huge cost—physically, financially, and psycho-spiritually."

With such a diverse background, Dr. Geffen is well versed in the strengths and weaknesses of different approaches to cancer. Among the first oncologists to blend Eastern and Western healing modalities, he has recently expanded his focus to include indigenous healing wisdom from the Northern and Southern Hemispheres, which he learned through his travels and explorations of ancient healing traditions of North and South America.

"There's a much deeper mystery involved in cancer than conventional Western medicine acknowledges. Science continues to pursue the reductionist dream that we can manipulate molecules and genes and find magic bullets for this disease. Although we've certainly made important progress, anyone working actively in this field recognizes what a huge mountain this is to climb. Cancer is very complex; it's multidimensional in nature. There are hundreds of different types with widely differing molecular and genetic profiles, and they arise in people of every imaginable size, shape, color, and background. Science will undoubtedly continue to make meaningful advances, but I'm doubtful that we'll find a single, magic bullet 'cure' for cancer.

"Then you look at Eastern traditions. I spent more than twenty years immersed in Eastern healing and spiritual paths. They certainly have much to offer, on many levels. But I also saw what I regard as the shadow of the Eastern traditions, especially the spiritual ones, which mirror the shadow of the Western traditions. The Eastern spiritual traditions tend to be more focused on consciousness and the mind than on emotions and feelings. They tend to be hierarchical, to honor the masculine more than the feminine, and they generally strive for the light rather than embrace the darker aspects of existence.

"Although Eastern traditions have certainly mastered a huge array of important meditation and other yogic practices, they often regard emotions as a distraction from the 'true path'—or even as 'afflictions' to be overcome—rather than as a portal to deep wisdom, self-understanding, and potential healing and transformation.

They rarely acknowledge the profound impact of the unconscious on the human experience.

"I've seen over and over again how people can spend thirty years eating well, exercising, practicing yoga and meditation, thinking positively, and cleansing and detoxifying the body, and still have many unhealed, unconscious, wounded parts of themselves that are impacting all aspects of their health, behavior, and well-being."

It sounded as though he was saying that, by themselves, neither Eastern nor Western practices hold the key for healing and wholeness. I asked him what does, and he replied, "First, I believe that it requires the best available conventional medicine, integrated with safe and effective complementary therapies and the wisdom of the Eastern traditions. If any alternative therapies are eventually proven effective, they should be included as well.

"I also think we should begin to more fully explore the ancient wisdom of the North and South American traditions, which are still largely unknown in our culture. I've been privileged to experience many traditional Native American ceremonies and to travel to South America and explore a variety of sacred plant medicines and other shamanic healing practices. I've been astonished by their strength, beauty, and power. I believe they hold immense promise for medicine in the postmodern world.

"Next, deep healing requires a psycho-spiritual perspective that embraces the mental, emotional, and spiritual dimensions of life, including the unconscious shadow and the wounded parts of the self that live in everyone. What's hard about this—for individuals and for our culture—is that it requires us to look inside and face the fragmented, disowned, and hurting parts of ourselves. This is rarely easy or comfortable. There are many potent ways to do this inner work that can make an enormous difference for people, including transpersonal and Jungian psychology and other powerful modalities, such as Holotropic Breathwork. I've been privileged to directly experience many of these, and

I actually became certified as a Holotropic Breathwork practitioner."

Other techniques that can accomplish similar types of psycho-spiritual healing include Voice Dialogue, Emotional Freedom Technique (EFT), Emotional Self-Management (ESM), Eye Movement Desensitization and Reprocessing (EMDR), PSYCH-K, and more. (See appendix.)

"We also need to acknowledge death as an intrinsic part of life. Open discussion about death is still a big taboo in our culture, particularly in the Western medical model, which tries to postpone death at all costs. But for genuine whole-person healing, it is imperative that we learn to navigate this part of the human journey with consciousness, grace, equanimity, and love.

"Finally, we need to understand cancer in a *multidimensional* way and coherently address the needs of body, mind, heart, *and* spirit. On the physical level, cancer is literally a part of us, our own cells run amok, mediated by genetic mutations and affected by diet, lifestyle, and environmental pollution.

On a more subtle level, it involves blockages of energy or life force called chi in the traditional Chinese medicine system, or *prana* in the Ayurvedic system.

"On the mental level, cancer brings up all kinds of thoughts and beliefs about health, illness, conventional versus nonconventional treatment options, doctors, healing, and life itself. These associations affect every decision people make about their care and can be deeply consequential. Some thoughts, beliefs, and decisions may be accurate and helpful, but others may be inaccurate, dysfunctional, or disempowering. And this can cause problems.

"Similarly, the mind assigns *meanings* to every event in our lives—including life with cancer—and these, too, can be either empowering or destructive. This is important to understand because the meanings that we consciously or unconsciously give to events impact not only our *experience* of life, but our *physiology* as well. This is occurring in every moment and at a profound level.

"On the emotional level, I believe that cancer may often reflect a physical manifestation of years of emotional pain, loneliness, or interpersonal dysfunction that so many people experience. It can represent wounded, hurting, repressed, or rejected parts of the self crying out for love and acceptance—and many of these parts are unconscious. If we don't welcome these parts into a conscious dialogue and aren't willing to face and feel the pain, sorrow, shame, or even rage that they hold, we miss an important opportunity to discover deeply hidden parts of ourselves and reclaim our wholeness as human beings. As life experience abundantly shows, if painful emotions are not expressed by the voice, sooner or later they will be expressed in the body. This is increasingly being understood scientifically, particularly by the fields of psychoneuroimmunology and psychosocial genomics."

As Dr. Geffen referenced these fragmented and abandoned parts of ourselves, Raven (my abandoned creative self described in chapter 1) came to mind. I feel fortunate that she showed herself so vividly and spoke so articulately about how she felt I had left her behind. Looked at objectively, however, it wasn't a sudden and unexpected visit. Indeed, I was on my third cancer diagnosis and had already spent a solid year looking deeply at myself in search of what was within me that had become the cancer. The fact that Raven appeared to me was certainly an act of grace, but it occurred also because I had been asking for the knowledge for years.

Dr. Geffen then quoted the thirteenth-century mystic poet, Rumi, who said, "That which haunts us will always find a way out. The wound will not heal until given witness. And the shadow that follows us is the way in."

He added, "This is one of my favorite quotes, because it so clearly expresses the fundamental truth that healing at the deepest levels begins with awareness. Becoming conscious of and giving witness to our emotional pain is the doorway to healing and becoming more whole.

"On a spiritual level, for many people, cancer may be a physical manifestation of the profound sense of separation that is endemic to our times and takes its toll on the body, mind, heart, and soul. This separation includes our estrangement from nature and other species; from our neighbors, families, and fellow humans on planet earth; and from the cosmos itself. It also includes separation from God, spirit, or whatever you call the mysterious, transcendent dimension of human existence that fundamentally underlies and interconnects all life.

"Honoring all these dimensions asks that we love and accept ourselves more fully than ever before and in a more intentional and authentic way. An essential component is to reflect this in our thinking and language; for example, we can move away from seeing cancer as a 'battle' to be won and move to seeing it as a healing journey to be fully lived."

I flashed on our cultural paradigm of declaring war on whatever threatens us. We have a war on terrorism, on drugs, on teenage pregnancy, and on cancer. The standard shock-and-awe approach clearly isn't winning any of our wars.

When I asked how he thinks these wounded parts come to be and to impact our health, he brought to light not only our physical, biological, social, and mental selves, but our spiritual and psychological selves as well. "Coming into human form and being born is not easy. The process of embodiment begins with a type of condensing down from a realm of absolute pure love, consciousness, and spirit—a dimension of existence described by mystics and sages for millennia. We then spend nine months growing and developing in a womb that is often not a Garden of Eden. That's because many of our parents, despite their best intentions, were neurotic, frightened, or had various kinds of dysfunctions. Most of our mothers were also living in a world of stress, processed foods, and environmental toxins, not to mention their own inner emotional pain and limitations. The impact of all this affects the growing fetus at a primordial, precognitive level.

"Then we go through the trauma of birth itself. Even when the birth is successful, it's an intense experience that can have enduring effects on one's psychology, personality, and perhaps even one's health."

According to Dr. Geffen, making it out of the womb is just the beginning. "Even if our parents were fundamentally kind, loving, and well adjusted, they were human, after all, and their capacity to give love unconditionally was limited. In every child's life, there comes a time when he or she gets criticized, shamed, or even abused in some way, physically or energetically, or the child may suffer the trauma of abandonment, neglect, or loss.

"In any event, the child believes that what occurred is her fault and begins to believe that there is something wrong with herself. As a result, a process of fragmentation begins. We create a false self, a mask, an identity or persona that many of us wear all our lives, believing it to be who we really are. The tragedy, of course, is that this false self often becomes a prison, cutting us off from our true selves, our life force, and, in many cases, the life path that would actually bring us the greatest joy and fulfillment.

"The impact of living with these wounds and deeply buried splits often eventually leads to a crisis of some kind, including physical or mental health challenges. We know, in fact, from highly credible studies that adverse childhood experiences—and the wounding and inner splits they cause—are directly correlated with a variety of significant health problems in adulthood.

"I'm not saying that these deeper issues are the primary, root cause of all cancers. However, in all my years as an oncologist, working with thousands of patients and loved ones, I have never encountered a situation where they were not clearly present. In any case, these issues are most always a rich, fertile source of potential healing and discovery for patients who have the courage and will to explore them.

"Of course, the genetic, dietary, lifestyle, and environmental components of cancer causation clearly play critical roles. After all, a fundamental dimension of our being is the physical one. But this is just one dimension of who we are, and to ignore the other dimensions is, I believe, shortsighted."

This made total sense to me and mirrored my own convictions about my own cancer. His suggestion about how to heal at the deepest levels also validated what I have come to know as true and what's worked for me.

He concluded by reiterating the need for committing to a life lived out of love and trust: "In the midst of intense, focused action, we can also respond with compassion, insight, humility, and love. This is important because the reflexive response to 'go to war' against cancer puts us in a warlike state inside, and it is difficult—if not impossible—to heal at the deepest levels with aggressive energy pervading our reality.

"So for example, along with using chemotherapy, radiation, surgery, diet and nutrition, exercise, massage, acupuncture, and a host of other powerful healing modalities, you can also engage in an inner exploration of parts of the self that may be unconscious and that are hurting and in pain. This cannot happen with the rational mind alone; it requires accessing emotions, feelings, and the unconscious. What messages are these cells trying to bring to consciousness? What wounds are longing for attention and healing?

"It's also incredibly valuable to reflect upon and clarify what is really most important to you: Why do you really want to live or not? What is the meaning and purpose of your life? What are your most important goals? Clarifying these questions can liberate enormous amounts of energy, so you can focus on what really matters most and heal at a deeper level."

"Finally, don't miss the opportunity to connect with and experience your spiritual self, that part of everyone that is untouched by the turbulent waves of existence."

Knowing who we really are, discovering that we are *not* separate from spirit or each other, and realizing that at the deepest level we already are and always have been free are among the many ideas echoed throughout Dr. Geffen's book. "Cancer, and why we get it, ultimately touches the mystery of the soul. Although we may hold a particular plan for our lives, or even our health, our souls may have a bigger agenda. For many people, the ordeal of cancer is the very thing, perhaps the *only* thing, that cracks open the armor of their 'false self' and opens a portal to an entirely new, more powerful, authentic, and expanded experience of life itself.

"I think the evolutionary imperative is to embrace it all. To evolve, we need to understand that life fundamentally includes many opposites and paradoxes: lightness and darkness, masculine and feminine, mind and emotions, body and spirit, joy and sorrow, health and illness, life and death. To grow and heal, we must learn to embrace them all within ourselves. To the degree that we do this, we become more conscious and can more fully heal ourselves. And in doing so, we help heal each other and the world."

Contact Information:

Geffen Visions International, Inc.

4450 Arapahoe Avenue, Suite 100
Boulder, Colorado 80303
Telephone: 303-444-6814
Fax: 303-444-6815
For more information visit geffenvisions
.com.

*Your vision will become clear only when
you look into your heart. Who looks
outside, dreams. Who looks inside,
awakens.*
CARL JUNG

EPILOGUE

The Cosmic Clothesline

I know now that the lives we live are really just an arena where our souls play out their evolution. We get excited about our jobs and cars, meeting the right mate, making enough money, going on trips, or fixing up the house. We talk well into the night about when and how many kids to have, or whether to have them at all. We get caught in the web of this drama or that, in a perpetual round of trying to get through one or the other. We give most of our attention to where our eyes are turned: outward. I now know that what goes on outside is the window dressing for what goes on inside.

The way we live our lives is a reflection of our personalities, but if we pay close attention, we can also tailor our choices so they reflect what calls from our souls. If we listen, every choice we make in this physical atmosphere can also reply to something hidden deep within the mystery of our soul's infinite journey. We have the ability—the responsibility, even—to satisfy not only everyday thirst, but also the desire that comes from or speaks to other worlds.

I see each of our souls as a clothesline and each one of our lives as another garment hanging from the line. The quality of our lives is told through our aesthetic, and the choices that we make shape the costume we call ourselves. The energy pulsating through the cosmic clothesline sustains, carries, guides, and animates us from lifetime to lifetime.

So what does this have to do with cancer? It's a simple image that reminds me we're hooked into something much bigger than the attire we call ourselves. The blessing of a cancer diagnosis is that it can catapult us into suddenly understanding how temporary the fabric is, thus nudging us to look deeper, forgive faster, say thank you more often, and love more devotedly. Cancer might just be a beckoning from our soul—a reminder of the need to attend to our deepest wounds, our most exhilarating dreams, our highest ambitions, and the sensitivity of both our physical and planetary environment.

The Centers for Disease Control keeps track of how many lives end because of cancer, but I wonder how many lives actually begin because of it. It surely launched the beginning of mine. My hope is that by reading this book, by opening to and embracing the beautiful truth of who you are—of who *we* are—and by releasing the grievances you have gripped for decades, or even just one day, you can count yourself among those who have healed.

Whether it's next week or in another fifty years, eventually the outfits we don will wither and fall away, but the source of all power never does. A piece of who we are—beyond the thread—remains in the promise of God's imperceptible design that there will always be another season.

How we fashion ourselves in the productions to come is largely decided by what inhabits our hearts right now.

I learned that a highly developed purpose and the will to live are among the prime raw materials of human

existence. I became convinced that these materials may well represent the most potent force within human reach.
NORMAN COUSINS

An Invitation

If you or a loved one has healed yourself of any disease and want to share your story with the public, please send a one-page synopsis to me along with contact information. I might want to use it in my next book!
Leigh@embracehealingcancer.com

APPENDIX

Publications by Authors Interviewed in This Book

Timothy Birdsall

How to Prevent and Treat Cancer with Natural Medicine: A Natural Arsenal of Disease-Fighting Tools for Prevention, Treatment, and Coping with Side Effects, from America's Foremost Authorities on Natural Medicine. With Michael Murray, Joseph E. Pizzorno, and Paul Reilly. New York: Riverhead Trade, 2003.

Barry Boyd, MD, FACP

The Cancer Recovery Plan: How to Increase the Effectiveness of Your Treatment and Live a Fuller, Healthier Life. With Marian Betancourt. New York: Avery, 2005.

Brenda Cobb

The Living Foods Lifestyle. Fort Bragg, CA: Living Light, 2002.

Nancy Deville

Death by Supermarket: The Fattening, Dumbing Down, and Poisoning of America. Fort Lee, NJ: Barricade Books, 2007.

Larry Dossey, MD

Be Careful What You Pray For: You Just Might Get It. New York: HarperOne, 1997.

Beyond Illness. Boston: Shambhala, 1984.

The Extraordinary Healing Power of Ordinary Things: Fourteen Natural Steps to Health and Happiness. New York: Three Rivers Press, 2006.

Healing Beyond the Body: Medicine and the Infinite Reach of the Mind. Boston: Shambhala, 2003.

Healing Words: The Power of Prayer and the Practice of Medicine. New York: HarperOne, 1993.

Meaning & Medicine. New York: Bantam, 1991. *The Power of Premonitions: How Knowing the Future Can Shape Our Lives.* New York: Dutton, 2009.

Prayer Is Good Medicine. New York: HarperOne, 1997.

Recovering the Soul: A Scientific and Spiritual Approach. New York: Bantam, 1989.

Reinventing Medicine: Beyond Mind-Body to a New Era of Healing. New York: HarperOne, 1999.

Space, Time & Medicine. Boston: Shambhala, 1982.

David Felten, MD, PhD

Psychoneuroimmunology. 3rd ed. San Diego, CA: Academic Press, 2001.

Jeremy Geffen, MD, FACP

The Journey Through Cancer: Healing and Transforming the Whole Person. New York: Three Rivers Press, 2006.

Charlotte Gerson

Healing the Gerson Way: Defeating Cancer and Other Chronic Diseases. With Beata Bishop. Carmel, CA: Totality Books, 2007.

James Gordon, MD

Comprehensive Cancer Care: Integrating Alternative, Complementary, and Conventional Therapies. New York: Perseus, 2001.

Manifesto for a New Medicine: Your Guide to Healing Partnerships and the

Wise Use of Alternative Therapies. New York: DaCapo, 1997.

Unstuck: Your Guide to the Seven-Stage Journey Out of Depression. New York: Penguin, 2009.

William B. Grant, PhD

"An estimate of premature cancer mortality in the United States due to inadequate doses of solar ultraviolet-B radiation, Cancer." 2002; 94:1867-75. (Twenty-six ISI citations).

"A multi-country ecologic study of risk and risk reduction factors for prostate cancer mortality." Eur. Urol. 2004; 45:371-9.

"A critical review of studies on vitamin D in relation to colorectal cancer." Nutr. Cancer. In press (accepted mid-February 2004).

"Geographic variation of prostate cancer mortality rates in the U.S.A.; implications for prostate cancer risk related to vitamin D"; Int. J. Cancer. (accepted Feb. 12, 2004).

Ryke Geerd Hamer, Med. Mag. Theol.

Summary of the New Medicine. N.p.: Amici di Dirk, 2000.

Abram Hoffer, MD, PhD

Healing Cancer: Complementary Vitamin & Drug Treatment. With Linus Pauling. Toronto: CCNM Press, 2004.

Orthomolecular Medicine for Everyone: Megavitamin Therapeutics for Families and Physicians. With Andrew W. Saul. Laguna Beach, CA: Basic Health Publications, 2008.

Putting It All Together: The New Orthomolecular Nutrition. New York: McGraw Hill, 1998.

User's Guide to Natural Therapies for Cancer Prevention & Control: Learn

How Diet and Supplements Can Help Prevent and Treat Cancer. Laguna Beach, CA: Basic Health Publications, 2004.

Vitamin C & Cancer: Discovery, Recovery, Controversy. With Dr. Linus Pauling. Gardena, CA: SCB Distributors, 2001.

The Vitamin Cure for Alcoholism: How to Protect Against and Fight Alcoholism Using Nutrition and Vitamin Supplementation. With Andrew W. Saul. Laguna Beach, CA: Basic Health Publications, 2009.

Laura Alden Kamm

Color Intuition: Master the Energy of Color for Higher Awareness, Extraordinary Perception, and Healing. Boulder, CO: Sounds True, 2009.

Intuitive Wellness: Using Your Body's Inner Wisdom to Heal. Hillsboro, OR: Beyond Words Publishing, 2006.

Peter Lambrou, PhD

Instant Emotional Healing: Acupressure for the Emotions. With George Pratt. New York: Broadway Books, 2006.

Self-Hypnosis: The Complete Guide to Better Health and Self-Change. With Brian Alman. London: Souvenir Press, 1993.

Bruce Lipton, PhD

The Biology of Belief: Unleashing the Power of Consciousness, Matter, and Miracles. Carlsbad, CA: Hay House, 2008.

Spontaneous Evolution: Our Positive Future (And a Way to Get There from Here). With Steve Bhaerman. Carlsbad, CA: Hay House, 2009.

The Wisdom of Your Cells: How Your Beliefs Control Your Biology. Boulder, CO: Sounds True, 2006. CDs.

Tullio Simoncini, MD

Cancer Is a Fungus: A Revolution in Tumor Therapy. Milan: Edizioni, 2007.

Books About Alternative Treatments and the Mind's Role with Cancer

Abrams, Donald, and Andrew Weil. *Integrative Oncology.* New York: Oxford University Press, 2009.

Anderson, Greg. *Cancer: 50 Essential Things to Do.* New York: Plume, 2009.

Anderson, Mike. *Healing Cancer from the Inside Out.* Glendale, CA: Ravediet, 2009.

Blaylock, Russell. *Natural Strategies for Cancer Patients.* New York: Kensington, 2003.

Block, Keith. *Life Over Cancer: The Block Center Program for Integrative*

Cancer Treatment. New York: Bantam, 2009.

Brown, Michael. *The Presence Process: A Healing Journey into Present Moment Awareness.* New York: Beaufort Books, 2005.

Carr, Kris. *Crazy Sexy Cancer Tips.* Guilford, CT: skirt!, 2007.

Cohen, Ken. *Qi Healing: Energy Medicine Techniques to Heal Yourself and Others.* Boulder, CO: Sounds True, 2000.

Greaves, Mel. *Cancer: The Evolutionary Legacy.* New York: Oxford University Press, 2002.

Griffin, G. Edward. *World Without Cancer: The Story of Vitamin B17.* Westlake Village, CA: America Media, 2010.

Hawkins, David. *Healing and Recovery.* West Sedona, AZ: Veritas Publishing Company, 2009.

Henderson, Bill. *Cancer-Free: Your Guide to Gentle, Non-Toxic Healing.* Bangor, ME: Booklocker.com, 2007.

Issells, Josef. *Cancer: A Second Opinion: A Look at Understanding, Controlling, and Curing Cancer.* Garden City Park, NY: Square One, 2005.

Kaufmann, Doug. *The Germ That Causes Cancer.* Rockwall, TX: Mediatrition, 2002.

Kinslow, Frank J. *The Secret of Instant Healing.* Sarasota, FL: Lucid Sea, 2008.

LeShan, Lawrence. *Cancer as a Turning Point: A Handbook for People with Cancer, Their Families, and Health Professionals.* New York: Plume, 1994.

Pierce, Tanya Harter. *Outsmart Your Cancer: Alternative Non-Toxic Treatments That Work.* Stateline, NV: Thoughtworks, 2009.

Rossman, Martin L. *Fighting Cancer from Within: How to Use the Power of Your Mind for Healing.* New York: Holt, 2003.

Siegel, Bernie, and Jennifer Sander. *Faith, Hope and Healing: Inspiring Lessons Learned from People Living with Cancer.* Hoboken, NJ: Wiley, 2009.

Simon, David. *Free to Love, Free to Heal: Heal Your Body by Healing Your Emotion.* Carlsbad, CA: Chopra Center Press, 2009.

_____. *Return to Wholeness: Embracing Body, Mind, and Spirit in the Face of Cancer.* New York: Wiley, 1999.

Trudeau, Kevin. *Natural Cures "They" Don't Want You to Know About.* Birmingham, AL: Alliance, 2005.

Books About Diet

Believeau, Richard, and Denis Gringas. *Foods to Fight Cancer: Essential Foods to Help Prevent Cancer.* New York: DK Adult, 2007.

Benzell, Philip B. *Alive and Well: One Doctor's Experience with Nutrition in the Treatment of Cancer Patients.*

Westlake Village, CA: American Media, 1994.

Campbell, T. Colin, and Thomas M. Campbell II. *The China Study: The Most Comprehensive Study of Nutrition Ever Conducted and the Startling Implications for Diet, Weight Loss, and Long-Term Health.* Dallas: BenBella, 2006.

Daniel, Kaayla T. *The Whole Soy Story: The Dark Side of America's Favorite Health Food.* Washington, DC: NewTrends, 2005.

Douglass, William Campbell, II. *The Raw Truth About Milk.* Miami: Rhino, 2007.

Plant, Jane A. *Your Life in Your Hands: Understanding, Preventing, and Overcoming Breast Cancer.* New York: St. Martin Press, 2000.

Pollan, Michael. *In Defense of Food: An Eater's Manifesto.* New York: Penguin, 2009.

_____. *The Omnivore's Dilemma: A Natural History of Four Meals.* New York: Penguin, 2007.

Servan-Schreiber, David. *Anti-Cancer: A New Way of Life.* New York: Viking, 2009.

Store, Diana. *Raw Food Works: Leading Experts Explain Why.* Holland: Raw Superfoods: 2008.

Vasey, Christopher. *The Acid-Alkaline Diet for Optimum Health: Restore Your Health by Creating pH Balance in Your Diet.* Rochester, VT: Healing Arts Press, 2006.

Weber, Karl. *Food Inc.: A Participant Guide: How Industrial Food Is Making Us Sicker, Fatter, and Poorer, and What You Can Do About It.* New York: PublicAffairs, 2009.

Weston, Andrew. *Nutrition and Physical Degeneration.* La Mesa, CA: Price Pottenger Nutrition, 2008.

Books and Audiobooks That Can Empower You Spiritually

Braden, Gregg. *The Divine Matrix: Bridging Time, Space, Miracles, and Belief.* Carlsbad, CA: Hay House, 2008.

_____. *The Spontaneous Healing of Belief: Shattering the Paradigm of False Limits.* Carlsbad, CA: Hay House, 2009.

_____. *Unleashing the Power of the God Code.* Carlsbad, CA: Hay House, 2005. CD.

Chödrön, Pema. *The Places That Scare You: A Guide to Fearlessness in Difficult Times.* Boston: Shambhala, 2005.

_____. *Unconditional Confidence: Instructions for Meeting Any Experience with Trust and Courage.* Boulder, CO: Sounds True, 2009. CD.

_____. *When Things Fall Apart: Heart Advice for Difficult Times.* Boston: Shambhala, 2002.

Chopra, Deepak, *The Soul of Healing Meditations.* New York: Rasa Music, 2001.

Chopra, Deepak, Marianne Williamson, and Debbie Ford. *The Shadow Effect: Illuminating the Hidden Power of Your True Self.* New York: HarperOne, 2010.

Hanh, Thich Nhat. *Peace Is Every Step: The Path of Mindfulness in Everyday Life.* New York: Bantam, 1992.

_____. *Taming the Tiger Within: Meditations on Transforming Difficult Emotions.* New York: Riverhead Trade, 2005.

_____. *True Love: A Practice for Awakening the Heart.* Boston: Shambhala, 2006.

Hay, Louise L., *Heal Your Body A–Z: The Mental Causes for Physical Illness and the Way to Overcome Them.* Carlsbad, CA: Hay House, 2001.

_____. *Love Yourself, Heal Your Life Workbook.* Carlsbad, CA: Hay House, 1990.

_____. *You Can Heal Your Life.* Carlsbad, CA: Hay House, 1984.

Hicks, Esther, and Jerry Hicks. *The Amazing Power of Deliberate Intent: Living the Art of Allowing.* Carlsbad, CA: Hay House, 2006.

_____. *The Astonishing Power of Emotions: Let Your Feelings Be Your Guide.* Carlsbad, CA: Hay House, 2008.

_____. *The Law of Attraction: The Basics of the Teachings of Abraham.* Carlsbad, CA: Hay House, 2006.

Katie, Byron. *Loving What Is: Four Questions That Can Change Your Life.* New York: Three Rivers Press, 2003.

_____. *Question Your Thinking, Change the World: Quotations From Byron Katie.* Carlsbad, CA: Hay House, 2007.

_____. *Who Would You Be Without Your Story? Dialogue with Byron Katie.* Carlsbad, CA: Hay House, 2008.

Lin, Chinyi, *Butterfly Guided Healing Meditation.* Eden Prairie, MN: Spring Forest Qigong, 2007, CD.

MacLeod, Ainslie. *The Transformation: Healing Your Past Lives to Realize Your Soul's Potential.* Boulder, CO: Sounds True, 2010.

Myss, Caroline. *Anatomy of the Spirit: The Seven Stages of Power and Healing.* New York: Three Rivers Press, 1997.

_____. *Defy Gravity: Healing Beyond the Bounds of Reason.* Carlsbad, CA: Hay House, 2009.

_____. *Why People Don't Heal and How They Can.* New York: Three Rivers Press, 1998.

Pert, Candace. *Molecules of Emotion: The Science Behind Mind-Body*

Medicine. New York: Simon & Schuster, 1999.

_____. *To Feel Good: The Science and Spirit of Bliss.* Boulder, CO: Sounds True, 2007. CD.

_____. *Your Body Is Your Subconscious Mind.* Boulder, CO: Sounds True, 2004. CD.

Tipping, Colin. *Finding Peace: Guided Practices for Radical Forgiveness.* Boulder, CO: Sounds True, 2010. CD.

_____. *Radical Forgiveness: A Revolutionary Five-Stage Process to Heal Relationships, Let Go of Anger and Blame, Find Peace in Any Situation.* Boulder, CO: Sounds True, 2009.

Tolle, Eckhart. *Finding Your Life's Purpose.* Vancouver: Eckhart Teachings Inc., 2009. CD.

_____. *Living a Life of Inner Peace.* Novato, CA: New World Library, 2004. CD.

_____. *The Power of Now: A Guide to Spiritual Enlightenment.* Novato, CA: New World Library, 2004.

_____. *Stillness Speaks.* Novato, CA: New World Library, 2003. Williamson, Marianne, *The Gift of Change: Spiritual Guidance for Living Your Best Life.* New York: HarperOne, 2006.

_____. *Meditations for a Miraculous Life.* Carlsbad, CA: Hay House, 2007. CDs.

_____. *A Return to Love: Reflections on the Principles of A Course in Miracles.* New York: Harper, 1996.

Books About the Politics of Cancer and Medicine

Angell, Marcia. *The Truth About the Drug Companies: How They Deceive Us and What to Do About It.* New York: Random House, 2005.

Brownless, Shannon. *Overtreated: Why Too Much Medicine Is Making Us Sicker and Poorer.* New York: Bloomsbury, 2008.

Davis, Devra. *The Secret History of the War on Cancer.* New York: Basic Books, 2009.

Ehrenclon, Martine. *Critical Condition: The Essential Hospital Guide to Get Your Loved One Out Alive.* Santa Monica, CA: Lemon Grove Press, 2008.

Epstein, Samuel S. *Cancer-Gate: How to Win the Losing Cancer War (Policy, Politics, Health and Medicine).* Amityville, NY: Baywood, 2005.

Faguet, Guy B. *The War on Cancer: An Anatomy of Failure, a Blueprint for the Future.* New York: Springer, 2008.

Lisa, P. Joseph. *The Assault on Medical Freedom.* Newburyport, MA: Hampton Roads, 1994.

Moss, Ralph. *The Cancer Industry: The Classic Exposé on the Cancer Establishment.* London: Equinox Press, 1996.

Proctor, Robert N. *Cancer Wars: How Politics Shapes What We Know and Don't Know About Cancer.* New York: Basic Books, 1996.

Links to Valuable People, Places, and Resources

Readers must take full responsibility for working with any of these doctors or centers. The author is not endorsing them; rather, she is relaying that they are available for your own consideration.

To find a doctor near you who practices Functional Medicine (which diagnoses and treats all conditions more naturally and holistically), go to functionalmedicine.org/findmyphysician/results.asp.

Dr. Barre Lando

Petrolia, CA
Tel: 707-629-3590
mattolevalleynaturals.com

Dr. E. Callebout

Nutricentre
Lower Ground Floor
7 Park Crescent
London W1B 1PF
United Kingdom
Tel: +44 (0)203 230 2040

Dr. Bertrand Babinet

Babinetics
1750 30th St., #104
Boulder, CO 80301
Tel: 303-823-0301
Fax: 303-823-5378
babinetics.com

Dr. Robin Terranella

Southwest Integrative Medicine
16429 N. Tatum Blvd., Ste. 200
Phoenix, AZ 85032
Tel: 480-285-9794
swintegrativemedicine.com

Alternative Cancer Website:
Provides a huge bank of information

ranging from the politics behind the FDA and World Health Organization to what cancer feeds on (sugar!) to all kinds of stuff you can do in the privacy of your own home. Beware, though: there is a dizzying amount of information. It may be best to read through it and consult with a practitioner who can help you weed out what's best for your situation. alternativehealth.co.nz/canceralternatives.htm

The Aviva Directory: Provides web links to a wide assortment of alternative treatments to different types of cancer .avivadirectory.com/index.php?search=cancer

CANCERactive: Britain's number-one holistic-cancer-information charity. It provides comprehensive cancer information on complementary therapies and alternative treatments.canceractive.com

Cancer Cure Foundation: Comprehensive website on alternative treatments throughout the United States, Mexico, and Europe. cancure.org/home.htm

Cancer Tutor: Offers all kinds of information on alternative clinics and tr eatments.cancertutor.com

I Cure Cancer: Testimonials of people who have healed themselves, plus articles that talk about the politics of cancer, different places to go, and doctors who treat cancer alternatively. icurecancer.com/#

Natural Standard: An international research collaboration that aggregates and synthesizes data on complementary and alternative therapies. naturalstanda rd.com

People Against Cancer: A grassroots, nonprofit, member-supported, public-benefit organization dedicated to "finding our members the most effective treatment for their type of cancer." peopleagainst cancer.net/default.asp

The Moss Report: A thorough and comprehensive resource for finding out the best treatment for your type of cancer, written by a respected medical writer. cancerdecisions.com/

Seattle Cancer Treatment and Wellness Center: Peopled with both medical and naturopathic oncologists, it offers mind-body programs, Chinese medicine, and more. seattlecancerwelln ess.com/

Shaw Regional Cancer Center: Located in Vail, Colorado, it conducts conventional treatment, but offers a holistic and mind-body approach. shaw cancercenter.com/

NOTES

Foreword

[1]   Marla Cone, "President's Cancer Panel: Environmentally Caused Cancers are 'Grossly Underestimated' and 'Needlessly Devastate American Lives,'" *Environmental Health News,* May 2010.

Chapter 1: My Story

[1]   Jean Shinoda Bolen, *Close to the Bone: Life-Threatening Illness and the Search for Meaning* (New York: Scribner, 1998).

[2]   Kris Carr, *Crazy Sexy Cancer Tips* (Guilford, CT: skirt!, 2007).

[3]   Candace B. Pert, *Molecules of Emotion: The Science Behind Mind-Body Medicine* (New York: Simon & Schuster, 1999).

[4]   Laura Alden Kamm, *Intuitive Wellness: Using Your Body's Inner Wisdom to Heal* (New York: Atria Books/Beyond Words, 2006).

[5]   Bruce Lipton, *The Biology of Belief: Unleashing the Power of Consciousness, Matter, and Miracles* (Carlsbad, CA: Hay House, 2008).

[6]   Myrtle Fillmore, *How to Let God Help You* (Unity Village, MO: Unity School of Christianity, 2006).

Chapter 2: Forgiveness

[1]   *Atlas of Cancer Mortality Rates in the United States, 1950–94* (National Cancer Institute, cancer.gov/atlasplus/new.html, 1999).

[2]   William B. Grant, "An Estimate of Premature Cancer Mortality in the US due to Inadequate Doses of Solar Ultraviolet-B Radiation," *Cancer* 94, no.6 (2002): 1867–1875.

[3]   William B. Grant and Cedric F. Garland, "The Association of Solar Ultraviolet B (UVB) with Reducing Risk of Cancer: Multifactorial Ecologic Analysis of Geographic Variation in Age-adjusted Cancer Mortality

Rates," *Anticancer Research* 26, no.4A (2006): 2687–2699.

Chapter 4: Authority

[1]   Ginny Fraser, "The Cancer Clinics, Cancer Treatment Centres and Cancer Specialists," *Integrated Cancer and Oncology News,*canceractive.com/cancer-active-page-link.aspx?n=2077.

[2]   Teresa Tsalaky, "Recovery from Colon Cancer—Diet, Herbs, Detoxification, and Cellular Regeneration," *Positive Health Magazine* no.91 (August 2003): 35–38.

Chapter 5: Energy

[1]   George Pratt and Peter Lambrou, *Instant Emotional Healing: Accupressure for the Emotions* (New York: Broadway, 2000).

Chapter 6: Belief

[1]   Ralph Moss, *The Cancer Industry: The Classic Expose on*

the Cancer Establishment (London: Equinox Press, 1996).

Chapter 8: Intuition

[1]   See chapter 1, note 4.

Chapter 10: Faith

[1]   Rita Klaus, *Rita's Story* (Orleans, MA: Paraclete Press, 1995).

[2]   Caryle Hirshberg and Marc Ian Barasch, *Remarkable Recovery: What Extraordinary Healings Tell Us About Getting Well and Staying Well* (Darby: PA: Diane, 1999).

Chapter 11: Dedication

[1]   Tullio Simoncini, *Cancer Is a Fungus: A Revolution in Tumor Therapy* (Milan: Edizioni, 2007)

[2]   Ian F. Robey, et. al., "Bicarbonate Increases Tumor pH and Inhibits Spontaneous Metastases," *Cancer Research* 69, no.6 (2009): 2260–2268.

Chapter 12: Trust

[1]   Colin Tipping, *Radical Forgiveness* (Boulder, CO: Sounds True, 2009).

[2]   Jeremy Geffen, *The Journey Through Cancer: Healing and Transforming the Whole Person* (New York: Three Rivers, 2006).

Reader's Guide

1. What's the first thing I should do upon getting a cancer diagnosis?

Take at least a day to yourself to absorb the shock. Doctors move fast when it comes to cancer, and on the same day of your diagnosis, you will probably be told what treatments they want you to do. It's important to take time for yourself so you can begin your journey with as much clarity of mind as possible. It's normal to feel everything from panic and terror to anger and despair. You may also go numb. It's a bumpy ride, and you need to find your own unique brand of strength to endure the trip. It may take time to find your strength, but you will.

You have a choice of what kind of treatments you do, so don't just assume you have to do what your doctors recommend. They will be urgent about getting started, but if you want to investigate alternatives, now is the time to do it. Most alternative treatments are more effective for those who have not yet been subjected to chemo or radiation. Your treatment choices will impact you enormously, so make sure you are in agreement with yourself about what you choose to do.

If you choose conventional treatment, speak to others who have had your type of cancer and ask what type of treatments they did. There is no standard that's used by doctors 100 percent of the time. Yes, they use chemo, but what kind and for how long? Yes, they use radiation, but which type, for how long, and how many grays (units or doses) did the treatment include?

More revealing than asking your doctor about side effects is to ask others who have had the treatment you plan to do. Patients are the experts on side effects, and it's wise to find out if they would do the treatment again or choose another path. But also keep in mind that everyone is different, and you may not experience side effects at all or in the same way.

Enlist whatever help you believe will support you—friends, prayer, meditation, or medication. Don't judge yourself for needing help. This is a biggie and the best opportunity in the world to learn that asking for help is OK. You don't have to go it alone.

If you decide to go the alternative route, see question 5 on page 417.

Educating yourself is empowering, and empowerment is an essential ingredient to your health and wholeness.

2. Should I get a second opinion?

That's entirely up to you. If you feel that a mistake was made with your diagnosis, the only thing that may make you feel certain is getting another opinion. If you are confident in the diagnosis, but uncertain about the treatment, get as many different opinions as you can so that you find a treatment with which you can align.

3. What if I don't like or trust my doctors?

Whether you're pursuing conventional or alternative treatments, if there is anything about your doctors that makes you feel uncomfortable (if they don't answer your questions adequately, if they are condescending or closed minded), you are not obligated to stay with them. You choose who you work with. If you do chemo or radiation, you'll be paying them and the treatment facility more money in a few months than most people make in several years, so you have the right to be in the company of people you trust.

One way to determine if your doctors are going to support your unique journey is to tell them you want the information they will relay to you framed positively. Remind them that their suggestions can create a ripple effect within you that can be constructive or destructive. If they don't understand the nocebo effect, explain it to them or find an article about it and pass it along to them. Chances are that you will be educating your doctor as much as they will be treating you.

Your doctors are not gods (even though they might think they are!). They are human beings and don't know everything. Be as communicative with them as possible. Most of them are doing the best they can and truly want to help. But again, they're working for you, and it's essential that you are comfortable with them.

Don't blame your doctors if treatments don't work. Neither conventional nor alternative choices work 100 percent of the time. You are as much an experiment as you are a patient. They don't know for a fact that the treatment they are giving will work or not. You must take responsibility for your experience and give yourself fully to the idea of healing, regardless of the type of treatment you choose.

4. If I choose to do conventional treatment (chemo, radiation, or surgery) what can I do to

help mitigate the side effects or make it easier to go through treatments?

First, ask your doctors if they are affiliated with any naturopathic or homeopathic doctors who can help with side effects. This is called integrative medicine, and, thankfully, it is becoming more common. If they do have an affiliation, follow their lead. If not, they will likely tell you not to do anything outside of their protocol because it could interfere with their treatments. If that's the case, they are probably out of their field of knowledge, and this is the only response they have.

If you feel strongly that complementary treatments could help (and they probably will), ask around. Interview health care professionals who have augmented cancer treatments before. The other option is to find an MD or clinic that offers integrative therapy. Even if you can't travel to that clinic and become its patient, you might be able to get good recommendations for what types and combinations of supplements could help. The clinic staff may even talk to your doctors and convince or educate them about what can help.

If your doctors are adamant and will not condone any complementary help, you have a decision to make. I went along with my docs and didn't do anything to help. It went against my instinct, and to this day, I believe I'm paying the price. One of my best friends chose not to tell her doctors, but worked very closely with a ND during her breast cancer treatments. Her MDs were amazed at how well she tolerated the chemo and how quickly she recovered. She took control of her situation, made sure the ND knew what he was doing, and empowered herself and her body with that choice.

If you go that route, do your homework. There are plenty of qualified practitioners who have worked in conjunction with allopathic cancer treatments.

5. If I choose not to do conventional treatments,

where do I begin to look for alternative treatments? How will I know if the doctor or treatment is legitimate?

Educate yourself about what's available. Start with the resources in this book. The web is chock full of information about alternative treatments, but be mindful that it's hard to discern which treatments, facilities, or doctors are ethical and successful with their approach. Ask people if they know of someone who has worked with an alternative practitioner. You may be surprised at how many have. Interview the doctors and ask for referrals of other patients. It is your responsibility to make a wise choice.

6. Should I change my diet, and if so, how and when?

My doctor says it won't help.

You "should" only do what you believe is in your best interest and what feels like an empowered decision. If changing your diet is a good fit for you, regardless of what your doctor says, go for it as soon as you can. Check out the many references in the appendix this book regarding the best anti-cancer diets. There is a growing body of evidence that food can either feed cancer or create an environment that is inhospitable for it. In addition to specific diets, learn about keeping your system as alkaline as possible. Science now shows that it's harder for cancer to live in an alkaline environment than an acidic one. Food intake largely determines your body's alkalinity.

If you decide to radically alter your diet, research the potential downsides of your choice. Veganism, for example, can lead to deficiencies in vitamin B12. It's easy to make that up through supplements, but without research, you may not know the downsides or what supplements can help.

Try not to be rigid with your diet. We live in a world where truly healthy food can be hard to find. Relax, trusting that when food choices are within your power, you will eat well. If food choices are not within your power, simply try to enjoy what's before you! Flexibility is key.

Keep in mind that your body chemistry will change over time. Be sensitive to what's best for it at any given time. Be open minded about adapting to your changing needs. Turn to a qualified health care professional to help you determine what your nutritional needs are at any given time.

7. Insurance pays for conventional treatment, but the paperwork is mind boggling. What can I do to simplify it?

Ask a loved one or friend to take over managing your health-related (or even all of your) bills. You will probably be inundated with bills not only from each of your doctors, but also from radiology and chemotherapy departments, the hospital itself, and so on. Don't ever assume that the charges are accurate. Someone needs to keep a close eye on all of it. Insurance companies are notorious for providing confusing or elusive statements. I was double billed by my hospital and later discovered that insurance wasn't covering eligible expenses.

You can also enlist the help of a professional advocate at your hospital, clinic, or cancer center, as well as at your insurance company. After months of trying to decode the mistakes that varying accounting departments had made—including at my insurance company—I finally found enormous relief through in-house advocates at each institution. They cost nothing to you; it's their job to help patients who are trying to struggle through the jungle of paperwork accounting departments create. Don't wait until you feel like you're drowning in confusion. Call the patient-services department and ask for help from the get-go. If they give you the run-around, keep pestering them. Be the squeakiest wheel you can be!

Meanwhile, keep your energy focused on healing rather than chasing down the right numbers on billing and insurance statements. Your friends and family want to help you through your journey, and this is a really great assignment to hand off to someone—preferably someone who is patient and good with numbers.

8. Why doesn't insurance generally pay for alternative treatment?

Ask your insurance company that question. Send them all the bills you know won't be covered. It gives them the signal that you are using alternative treatments and they should get on board. Maybe someday they will.

9. What should I do if I find a good alternative doctor,

but don't have enough money to do the protocol?

Ask the doctor if there's a payment plan or some type of scholarship fund that can help. Some doctors will work with you; others won't. You can also ask a friend to start an alternative-healing fund where your friends and family can donate money for treatments. My friend did that for me, and I had a steady balance of about $5,000 for several months. It enabled me to pursue important complementary treatments. A fund such as this may not cover everything, but can help.

At one point, I was willing to sell some old family jewelry to raise money for alternative care. It was a hard choice because the jewelry had been in my family for generations. But after some soul searching, I realized that the jewelry would be meaningless if I was too sick to appreciate it, and that my health was more important. Fortunately, I found another way to pay for the treatment and didn't end up selling the heirlooms. The point is, if you own something of value, consider selling it. Weigh the material value of your item against your peace of mind and well-being. Selling it may be just what you need to provide the treatment you want.

Finally, if you have a wealthy friend or relative, ask for their help. All they can say is no. But you never know; they just might say yes!

10. Is it important to engage in the relationship between the mind and body regardless of what treatment I choose?

If you want to heal on every level, yes, it's important.

A cancer diagnosis is typically accompanied by fear. You'll need to go through all the normal feelings associated with a diagnosis; accept and express them. But eventually, you can pay attention to how thoughts trigger feelings. You'll quickly discover that negative thoughts provoke uncomfortable feelings and positive thoughts inspire upbeat ones. Feelings and emotions have an impact on your cells. Dwelling in the attributes of fear (anger, resentment, hopelessness, despair, and so on) can be unhealthy, while dwelling in the attributes of love (acceptance, forgiveness, compassion, hope, gratitude, and so on) can boost your immune system and contribute to improved health. As you train yourself to focus on more positive thoughts, be assured that bouts of negative emotions will not be harmful; they're normal. When you get stuck in negativity, that's when emotions can eventually become toxic to your body.

Do what you can to focus on healing rather than on cancer. The more energy, thought, and emotion you put into the idea that you "have cancer," the harder it will be to believe you don't have to have cancer, that you can heal, and that you can fully restore your health again. Go through the emotions that surface, but don't get stuck in anything less than going for perfect health. Create an intention to be healthy. Do whatever's necessary to recalibrate your mind so that you focus and dedicate yourself to healing, not disease.

Read what you can about how the mind and body are one. There is a good list of books in the appendix to get you started. The good news is that this stuff is not only really interesting, it's a big part of how to help rid yourself of cancer and be empowered in all aspects of your life.

11. I agree that our thoughts and emotions impact our cells and I can even identify how the negative emotions I've been feeling may have contributed to getting cancer. But right now, I'm so scared and feel so confused and powerless that I can't even begin to change

my thoughts and emotions to more positive ones.

This journey is played out one step at a time. Sometimes that means one day at a time, sometimes it means one hour at a time. It's good to acknowledge that there will be dark, horrible days. That's part of the program. Those days are also what can inspire you to look for relief.

The most important thing you can do when you're feeling scared and powerless is to love yourself. Whenever possible, find love. Dwell in it. Bathe in it. Allow the power of love to guide you. Love is the governing energy of the universe and can heal.

12. What can I do beyond exploring the relationship between my thoughts and emotions to access my

inner healing power? When should I start?

To access the healer within, you must dig deep. You will have to release a lifetime of old habits and negative thinking. You will have to immerse yourself in the power of love—self-love. Love of your body. Love of your life. Love of the journey. It takes discipline and fortitude that few other journeys require.

The sooner you access the healing energy within, the better. Here's a list of just a few ways you can create an environment that awakens your inner healer:

- Inundate yourself with positive affirmations, books, images, and people.
- Read everything you can about self-healing.
- Pamper yourself with small indulgences that will support your feelings of goodwill and joy.
- Be kind to yourself no matter what; accept that you are on a roller

coaster and there will be rough days.

- Believe in yourself. Believe in healing.
- Find peace in every day.
- Pray or meditate every day.
- Eat well.
- Create a protective bubble around yourself that keeps you insulated from all the negativity of the world. Avoid gossip, the news, dark movies, violent television shows, or books that feature human beings at their worst.
- Watch funny movies or those that highlight the best of humankind. Listen to comedy. Read funny or uplifting books. There are millions of them.
- Ask for help. Accept it with gratitude.
- Spend at least two minutes every day voicing out loud what you are thankful for.
- Learn about creative visualization and do it every day.
- Be honest about your journey. Don't sugarcoat the bad days. They suck. Yell and scream. Allow yourself to

have abysmal moods, but recover as quickly as you can, knowing that you are on the path of healing.

- See a therapist, hypnotherapist, or energy healer to make sure your conscious and/or subconscious mind is on board with the treatments you have chosen.
- Forgive everyone you know for everything they've ever done to you. Forgive yourself for everything you've ever done to them or to yourself.
- Be still and listen to what's inside—every day.
- Love yourself. If you don't know how to, read books about it and learn. Loving yourself is essential to this journey. It's also essential to healing.
- Breathe deeply as often as you need to.
- Seek out and be inspired by other people's stories. There are many.
- Do whatever makes you joyful. Sing. Dance. Be with babies and animals. Walk in nature. Sit in the sun. Take a vacation. Tell people

you love them. Ask them to tell you the same.

- If you can, if you have the energy, and only if you want to, be of service to someone else. Don't feel guilty if the time isn't right. Acknowledge how you give of yourself in your everyday life.
- Think of cancer as a big, fat wake-up call to live your life differently and better than you ever have before. Take this experience and turn it into a blessing.
- Focus on what you want. Go for it.
- Trust that you are being guided. Trust yourself. Trust life. Trust God.

13. What if deep down inside I don't believe that our thoughts and emotions can influence our healing?

You can believe whatever you want. That's the product of free will.

Read the chapter in this book about belief (Chapter 6). It will help you to understand that whatever you believe is what shapes your life experience. As always, the choice is yours.

14. Some of my friends and family judge me when I tell them that that I'm going to embrace my role in why the cancer came about, release the things that aren't good for me, and heal. I need their support through all this, but they don't believe in the path I'm taking. Should I join a support group?

Don't feel obligated to tell everyone you know about your choices. It's fine to be selective. You have the right to be as private or as public as you want. There are no rules to this game; you make them up as you go along. The most important thing is for you to feel good and right about the decisions you make, including who you include in your healing journey.

There's nothing you can do about other people's judgments. Focus on loving them regardless of whether or not they understand or approve of your choices. Do what you can to be in the company of those who support you and upon whom you can rely for reassurance and strength.

If you join a support group, make sure it's one that helps you believe in your healing rather than one where people remain fixed on having cancer, being "survivors," and "beating cancer." Although they can be helpful, they take a different track than what this book suggests. Perhaps a group of spiritually mind people who believe in the infinite possibilities of healing would be a good place to start.

15. Do I have to believe in God to activate the healing energy inside?

Absolutely not. There are many people who heal themselves who don't believe in God. Read Jeff's story in this book (Chapter 5, page 148) for a great example. Whether you believe in God or not, you have the God-given power to heal.

16. I've had to let some of my friendships go because they aren't healthy for me. But I feel like I've hurt people in the process. What can I do to feel better?

Engage in self-forgiveness. Forgive them. Dedicate a meditation to sending them loving energy. Acknowledge yourself for being true to yourself, your healing, and your lasting well-being. If the relationships weren't healthy for you, they probably weren't healthy for the other people either. Think of the separation as a liberation for all of you, even if you're the only one who knows it. If necessary, talk to a therapist or friend about it. Do whatever is necessary to release the guilt.

17. The more I heal on every level, the more I'm changing. Not everyone likes it or understands it. Is this normal?

Who knows what normal is? People change all of the time. If the changes you've undergone make you feel freer and happier and more loving, then you can be at peace. You can share your newfound freedom with those people you love and want in your life. Coming from a place of love will likely inspire more love within them.

18. I'm finished with my (alternative or conventional) treatments and am cancer free, but I find myself falling back into old habits that probably aren't good for

me. How can I stay on track?

Practice. Keep doing whatever you did to heal. Read the suggestions in the answer to question 12 and do them for as long as it takes to anchor in the change. The process never ends!

19. I'm finished with treatments. I've done my best to clean out my body and my mind, but the cancer came back. Am I doing something wrong?

No, you have done nothing wrong. You are in charge of the quality of your life and the choices you make around what happens to you. But we possess little awareness and virtually no control over of what our souls have crafted. There is a bigger story playing out, and in some ways, we're just along for the ride. We have great power in determining how smooth or bumpy the ride will be. But our soul's journey may not take us where we think we want to go; the destination isn't always something we can dictate. Still, we can keep our intentions clear and our lives purposeful, no matter what transpires. Healing is not a guarantee that we become cancer free, but the process of healing frees us so that the lives we live are brimming over with love and peace. There is no greater place to be than that.

About the Author

Leigh Fortson's interest in wellness began long before her own health was challenged. For the past two decades, she has written about alternative medicine, nutrition, childhood obesity, and end-of-life issues for mass market publications and various magazines. Leigh is also an award-winning playwright and has enjoyed productions of her short plays across the country. Leigh is available for speaking engagements and for consulting with people about their health matters at e mbracehealingcancer.com. Today she has a clean bill of health and lives in western Colorado with her husband of many years, two mesmerizing children, and five pets.

About Sounds True

Sounds True is a multimedia publisher whose mission is to inspire and support personal transformation and spiritual awakening. Founded in 1985 and located in Boulder, Colorado, we work with many of the leading spiritual teachers, thinkers, healers, and visionary artists of our time. We strive with every title to preserve the essential "living wisdom" of the author or artist. It is our goal to create products that not only provide information to a reader or listener, but that also embody the quality of a wisdom transmission.

For those seeking genuine transformation, Sounds True is your trusted partner. At SoundsTrue.com you will find a wealth of free resources to support your journey, including exclusive weekly audio interviews, free downloads, interactive learning tools, and other special savings on all our titles.

To listen to a podcast interview with Sounds True publisher Tami Simon and author Leigh Fortson, please visit Soun dsTrue.com/bonus/Leigh_Fortson_Embrace.

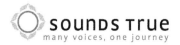

Back Cover Material

"A must read if you or someone you love is dealing with cancer."
—MARTIN L. ROSSMAN, MD, AUTHOR OF *FIGHTING CANCER FROM WITHINC*

"Leigh Fortson has journeyed through territory where many will eventually go—the land of cancer. She has returned a very wise woman whose insights will empower anyone with this diagnosis. The stories and interviews in *Embrace, Release, Heal* are full of hope and meaning. I hope this inspiring book is widely read."
—LARRY DOSSEY, MD, AUTHOR OF *THE SCIENCE OF PREMONITIONS*

"At last! In *Embrace, Release, Heal* we have testimony that proves that the healing of cancer involves the psychosomatic network of energy, mind, and spirit. Leigh Fortson is so courageous, not only for surviving her ordeal but also for standing up to the cancer docs who were shocked by the

independent thinking and bold decisions that led to her recovery. This is a gripping, compassionate, and well-researched exposé that I hope will revolutionize cancer treatment in this country."
 —CANDACE PERT, PHD, AUTHOR OF
  MOLECULES OF EMOTION

***

 After her third cancer diagnosis in three years, Leigh Fortson was given few options by her doctors and little hope for a bright future. For weeks, she mourned the life she thought she was losing—until she was introduced to an idea that changed everything: Our thoughts and emotions influence every cell in our body. This revelation gave her the hope that would begin her journey to becoming cancer free and more joyful than she'd ever been before. *Embrace, Release, Heal* shares her inspirational story and the fruits of her research in one empowering book. Created to help anyone whose life has been affected by cancer, this in-depth resource offers interviews with both allopathic and integrative medical experts; remarkable accounts from people who transcended "terminal cancer" and are now thriving; snapshots of progressive treatment techniques; and insights into other key factors that can affect well-being—including thoughts, emotions, and diet.

LEIGH FORTSON has coauthored and edited numerous books about health, nutrition, and alternative medicine. She spent decades learning about and practicing healthy lifestyle habits and was shocked to find out in 2006 that she had cancer. Today she has a clean bill of health and lives in Colorado with her family.

CPSIA information can be obtained
at www.ICGtesting.com
Printed in the USA
LVHW011931160322
713569LV00005B/219